Obsessive-Compulsive Disorder in Adults

About the Authors

Jonathan S. Abramowitz, PhD, is Professor and Director of the Clinical Psychology Doctoral Program at the University of North Carolina (UNC) at Chapel Hill. He is also a North Carolina licensed psychologist with a diplomate from the American Board of Professional Psychology. Dr. Abramowitz is an international expert on anxiety and OCD and has published 20 books and over 350 research articles and book chapters. He is the founder and former editor of the *Journal of Obsessive-Compulsive and Related Disorders*. Dr. Abramowitz has served as President of the Association for Behavioral and Cognitive Therapies.

Ryan J. Jacoby, PhD, is Assistant Director of the Center for OCD and Related Disorders in the Department of Psychiatry at the Massachusetts General Hospital in Boston and Assistant Professor at Harvard Medical School. Her clinical and research interests are focused on the nature and treatment of OCD and related disorders, and she has authored over 40 scientific publications on these topics. She has received funding for her work from the National Institute of Mental Health and the International OCD Foundation and serves on the editorial board of several academic journals.

Advances in Psychotherapy – Evidence-Based Practice

The basic objective of this series is to provide therapists with practical, evidence-based treatment guidance for the most common disorders seen in clinical practice – and to do so in a reader-friendly manner. Each book in the series is both a compact "how-to" reference on a particular disorder for use by professional clinicians in their daily work and an ideal educational resource for students as well as for practice-oriented continuing education.

The most important feature of the books is that they are practical and easy to use: All are structured similarly and all provide a compact and easy-to-follow guide to all aspects that are relevant in real-life practice. Tables, boxed clinical "pearls," marginal notes, and summary boxes assist orientation, while checklists provide tools for use in daily practice.

Continuing Education Credits

Psychologists and other healthcare providers may earn five continuing education credits for reading the books in the *Advances in Psychotherapy* series and taking a multiple-choice exam. This continuing education program is a partnership of Hogrefe Publishing and the National Register of Health Service Psychologists. Details are available at https://www.hogrefe.com/us/cenatreg

The National Register of Health Service Psychologists is approved by the American Psychological Association to sponsor continuing education for psychologists. The National Register maintains responsibility for this program and its content.

Advances in Psychotherapy – Evidence-Based Practice, Volume 31

Obsessive-Compulsive Disorder in Adults

2nd edition

Jonathan S. Abramowitz
Department of Psychology and Neuroscience, University of North Carolina at Chapel Hill, NC

Ryan J. Jacoby
Massachusetts General Hospital, Harvard Medical School, Boston, MA

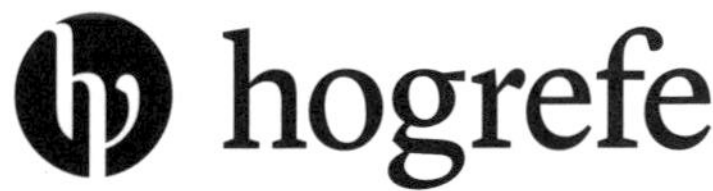

Library of Congress Cataloging in Publication information for the print version of this book is available via the Library of Congress Marc Database under the Library of Congress Control Number 2025945064

Library and Archives Canada Cataloguing in Publication
Title: Obsessive-compulsive disorder in adults / Jonathan S. Abramowitz, Department of Psychology and Neuroscience, University of North Carolina at Chapel Hill, NC, Ryan J. Jacoby, Massachusetts General Hospital, Harvard Medical School, Boston, MA.
Names: Abramowitz, Jonathan S., author. | Jacoby, Ryan J., author.
Series: Advances in psychotherapy--evidence-based practice ; v. 31.
Description: 2nd edition. | Series statement: Advances in psychotherapy--evidence-based practice ; volume 31 | Includes bibliographical references.
Identifiers: Canadiana (print) 20250257289 | Canadiana (ebook) 20250265435 | ISBN 9780889376076 (softcover) | ISBN 9781616766078 (PDF) | ISBN 9781613346075 (EPUB)
Subjects: LCSH: Obsessive-compulsive disorder. | LCSH: Obsessive-compulsive disorder—Treatment. | LCSH: Obsessive-compulsive disorder—Case studies. | LCSH: Evidence-based psychiatry. | LCGFT: Case studies.
Classification: LCC RC533 .A29 2025 | DDC 616.85/227—dc23

www.hogrefe.com

Publishing Offices
USA: Hogrefe Publishing Corporation, 44 Merrimac St., Newburyport, MA 01950
Phone 978 255 3700; E-mail customersupport@hogrefe.com
EUROPE: Hogrefe Publishing GmbH, Merkelstr. 3, 37085 Göttingen, Germany
Phone +49 551 99950 0, Fax +49 551 99950 111; E-mail publishing@hogrefe.com

Sales & Distribution
USA: Hogrefe Publishing, Customer Services Department, 30 Amberwood Parkway, Ashland, OH 44805
Phone 800 228 3749, Fax 419 281 6883; E-mail customersupport@hogrefe.com
UK: Hogrefe Ltd, Hogrefe House, Albion Place, Oxford, OX1 1QZ
Phone +44 186 579 7920; E-mail customersupport@hogrefe.co.uk
EUROPE: Hogrefe Publishing, Merkelstr. 3, 37085 Göttingen, Germany
Phone +49 551 99950 0, Fax +49 551 99950 111; E-mail publishing@hogrefe.com

Other Offices
CANADA: Hogrefe Publishing Corporation, 82 Laird Drive, East York, Ontario, M4G 3V1
SWITZERLAND: Hogrefe Publishing, Länggass-Strasse 76, 3012 Bern

Printed and bound in the USA

ISBN 978-0-88937-607-6 (print) • ISBN 978-1-61676-607-8 (PDF) • ISBN 978-1-61334-607-5 (EPUB)
https://doi.org/10.1027/00607-000

Dedication

To our parents: Ferne and Leslie Abramowitz; Doug and Jennie Jacoby.

Acknowledgments

We are indebted to a large group of people, including series editor Danny Wedding and Robert Dimbleby of Hogrefe, for their invaluable guidance and suggestions. The pages of this book echo with the clinical wisdom we have acquired through direct and indirect learning from masters of the science and art of psychological theory and intervention, including Joanna Arch, Donald Baucom, David A. Clark, Michelle Craske, Edna Foa, Martin Franklin, Michael Kozak, Jack Rachman, Paul Salkovskis, and Michael Twohig.

We dedicate this book to our clients and research participants who come to us seeking help and, in the face of uncertainty, find the courage to approach what they fear and give up their compulsive behaviors so that they can achieve a better quality of life. They believe in us, confide in us, challenge us, and educate us.

Contents

Preface

This book describes the conceptualization, assessment, and psychological treatment of *obsessive-compulsive disorder* (OCD) in adults, using empirically supported *cognitive behavior therapy* (CBT) interventions. The centerpiece of this approach is *exposure and response prevention* (ERP), a well-studied tandem of CBT techniques derived from learning theory accounts of OCD. The delivery of ERP is also informed by the fields of cognitive therapy, *acceptance and commitment therapy* (ACT), couples therapy, and inhibitory learning. We assume the reader will have basic knowledge and training in the delivery of psychotherapeutic interventions, yet not necessarily be a specialist in OCD. This book is for mental health professionals and trainees wishing to learn therapeutic strategies for managing OCD effectively in day-to-day clinical practice.

The book is divided into five chapters. The first describes the clinical phenomenon of OCD differentiating it from other problems with similar characteristics and outlining scientifically based diagnostic and assessment procedures. Chapter 2 reviews leading theoretical approaches to the development and maintenance of OCD, and their treatment implications. In Chapter 3, we present a framework for conducting an initial assessment of OCD and for deciding whether a particular client is a candidate for the treatment program in this volume. Methods for explaining the diagnosis of OCD and introducing the treatment program to clients are incorporated. Chapter 4 presents the details of how to conduct effective ERP for OCD. There are numerous case examples and transcripts of in-session dialogs to illustrate the treatment procedures. All case examples are based on composites of clients and our clinical experiences but do not represent any specific individual. The chapter also reviews the scientific evidence for the efficacy of this program and discusses how to identify and surmount a number of common obstacles to successful outcomes. Finally, Chapter 5 includes a series of case examples describing the treatment of various sorts of OCD symptoms (contamination concerns, fears of responsibility for harm, etc.). A variety of forms and client handouts for use in treatment appear in the book's Appendix.

OCD is a highly heterogeneous problem. Some clients experience fears of germs and contamination, while others have recurring, unwanted anxiety-evoking ideas of acting in ways that are wholly inconsistent with their values or character (e.g., using racial slurs or deliberately running into pedestrians while driving). Still others experience senseless but distressing doubts about unsolvable or existential questions (e.g., "how do I know I'm really in love," "what if my existence is just a dream?"). It is rare to see two individuals with completely overlapping symptoms. Thus, we provide a multicomponent approach that guides the clinician in structuring treatment to meet individual clients' needs. In this book you will find practical clinical information and illustrations, along with supporting didactic materials for both you and your clients.

1

Description

1.1 Terminology

Obsessive-compulsive disorder (OCD) has traditionally been considered an anxiety-related disorder. In the *Diagnostic and Statistical Manual of Mental Disorders*, 5th edition, text revision (DSM-5-TR; American Psychiatric Association [APA], 2022), it became the flagship diagnosis of the *obsessive-compulsive and related disorders* (OCRDs), a category of conditions with putatively overlapping features (see Section 1.5).

1.2 Definition

Definition of obsessions and compulsions

OCD is defined in the DSM-5-TR by the presence of obsessions and compulsions that are time-consuming, typically taking up an hour or more each day, and cause significant distress or impairment in social, occupational, or other important areas of functioning. *Obsessions* are repetitive and persistent thoughts, images, or doubts that are experienced as intrusive and unwanted, cause distress such as anxiety, shame, guilt, or doubt, and are not simply worries about real-life problems (e.g., unlike in generalized anxiety disorder). Individuals with obsessions typically attempt to ignore, suppress, or neutralize them with other thoughts or actions.

Although highly specific to the individual, obsessions typically concern the following themes: aggression and violence, responsibility for causing physical or emotional harm (e.g., by making a mistake), contamination, sex, religion, the need for exactness or completeness, and serious illnesses (e.g., cancer). Most people diagnosed with OCD experience multiple types of obsessions. Examples of common and uncommon obsessions appear in Box 1.

Compulsions are repetitive behaviors (e.g., handwashing) or mental acts (e.g., counting, praying) that a person feels driven to perform in response to an obsession or according to rigid rules. These actions are intended to prevent or reduce distress or prevent some dreaded event but are excessive or not realistically connected to the feared outcomes.

As with obsessions, rituals are highly individualized. Examples of behavioral (overt) rituals include repetitious handwashing, checking (e.g., locks, the stove), and repeating routine actions (e.g., going through doorways).

Examples of mental rituals include excessive prayer, repeating special phrases or numbers to oneself to neutralize obsessional fear, and mentally analyzing intrusive thoughts. Box 2 presents examples of some common and uncommon compulsive rituals.

People with OCD vary in their level of insight, ranging from good or fair to poor or absent, and this may fluctuate over time or depending on the specific obsessional theme. In some cases, OCD can co-occur with tics, in which distressing somatic sensations – such as physical discomfort – are temporarily relieved by movements or vocalizations.

Box 1
Examples of Common and Uncommon Obsessions

Common obsessions

- The idea that one is contaminated from dirt, germs, animals, body fluids, bodily waste, or household chemicals
- Doubts that one is (or may become) responsible for harm, bad luck, or other misfortunes such as fires, burglaries, awful mistakes, and injuries (e.g., car accidents)
- Unacceptable sexual ideas (e.g., of molesting a child)
- Unwanted violent impulses (e.g., to attack a helpless person)
- Unwanted sacrilegious thoughts (e.g., of desecrating a place of worship)
- Need for order, symmetry, completeness
- Fears of certain numbers (e.g., 13, 666), colors (e.g., red), or words (e.g., murder)

Uncommon obsessions

- Fear of having an abortion without realizing it
- Fear that not being able to remember events fully means they didn't occur
- Fear of that one's mind is contaminated by thoughts of unethical situations
- Fear of contamination from a geographic region
- Distressing preoccupations with bodily processes (e.g., breathing, blinking, swallowing, eye contact)
- Existential preoccupations about the meaning of life or one's own existence (e.g., "Am I real?")

Box 2
Examples of Common and Uncommon Compulsive Rituals

Common rituals

- Washing one's hands 40 times per day or taking multiple (lengthy) showers
- Repeatedly cleaning objects or vacuuming the floor
- Returning several times to check that the door is locked
- Placing items in the "correct" order to achieve "balance"
- Retracing one's steps
- Rereading or rewriting things to prevent mistakes
- Calling relatives or "experts" to ask for reassurance

- Thinking the word "healthy" to counteract hearing the word "cancer"
- Repeated and excessive confessing of one's "sins"
- Repeating a prayer until it is said perfectly

Uncommon rituals

- Having to touch (with equal force) the right side of one's body after being touched on the left side
- Having to look at certain points in space in a specified way
- Having to mentally rearrange letters in sentences to spell out comforting words
- Having to blink in a way that feels "just right"
- Excessive list making or digital cataloging of information

1.2.1 Avoidance

Avoidance functions to reduce discomfort or prevent perceived harm

People with OCD often use avoidance behaviors as a strategy for evading situations, objects, or thoughts that trigger obsessions or provoke anxiety. Avoidance functions as a coping mechanism aimed at reducing or controlling discomfort or preventing perceived harm associated with obsessions. Avoidance can be overt (e.g., refraining from using public restrooms) or more subtle (e.g., procrastination, distraction).

1.2.2 Insight

Individuals vary in terms of their insight into the senseless of their symptoms

People with OCD show a range of *insight* into the validity of their obsessions and compulsions – some acknowledge that their obsessions are unrealistic (i.e., acknowledging that their feared consequences are unlikely to occur and that they perform their compulsions because "it's better to be safe than sorry" or simply because it reduces their distress), while others are more firmly convinced (approaching delusional intensity) that their symptoms are rational. To accommodate this parameter of OCD, the DSM-5-TR includes specifiers to denote whether the person has (a) good or fair, (b) poor, or (c) no insight into the senselessness of their OCD symptoms. Often, the degree of insight varies within a person across time, situations, and across types of obsessions. For example, someone might have good insight into the senselessness of their obsessional thoughts about violence yet have poor insight regarding fears of contamination from chemicals.

1.2.3 Tics

DSM-5-TR also includes a specifier to distinguish between people with OCD with and without tics (or a history of a tic disorder). Whereas in OCD, obsessions lead to a negative *emotional* (affective) state such as anxiety or fear, tics are characterized by a distressing *sensory* (somatic) state such as physical discomfort in specific body parts (e.g., face) or a diffuse psychological distress or tension (e.g., "in my head"). This sensory discomfort is then relieved by motor responses (e.g., head twitching, eye blinking). (More details regarding differential diagnosis of OCD vs. tics/Tourette's disorder are reviewed in Section 1.5.3)

1.2.4 OCD From an Interpersonal Perspective

OCD commonly has an interpersonal component

The previous description highlights the experience of OCD from the individual's perspective. Yet OCD commonly has an interpersonal component that may negatively impact close relationships, such as that with a parent, sibling, spouse, or romantic partner (Abramowitz et al., 2013). This component may be manifested in two ways. First, a partner or spouse (or other close friend or relative) might inadvertently be drawn to help with or accommodate the performing of compulsive rituals and avoidance behavior out of a desire to show care or concern for the individual with OCD (e.g., to help reduce anxiety). Second, OCD symptoms may lead to arguments and other forms of conflict within these relationships.

Symptom Accommodation

Accommodation occurs when a loved one (a) participates in the client's rituals (e.g., answers reassurance-seeking questions, performs cleaning and checking behaviors for the client), (b) helps with avoidance strategies (e.g., avoids places deemed "contaminated" by the client), or (c) helps to resolve or minimize problems that have resulted from the client's OCD symptoms (e.g. making excuses for the person's behavior, supplying money for special soaps). Accommodation might occur at the request (or demand) of the individual with OCD or it might be voluntary and based on the desire to show care and concern by reducing the distress of the individual with OCD. The following vignette illustrates accommodation:

> Avery adores her dog, Sadie, a gentle golden retriever who has been her loyal companion for years. Recently, Avery has been plagued by intrusive thoughts of accidentally harming Sadie. These thoughts terrify her, leading her to avoid activities like cooking, where she fears a knife might slip and hurt Sadie. She refuses to watch movies or shows that depict violence and insists on rearranging her furniture to avoid any accidental collisions that could harm her pet. Avery's partner, Cameron, does everything possible to ensure that sharp objects are safely stored away, avoids discussing any potentially upsetting topics related to pets, and even rearranges their daily routines to minimize any perceived risks to Sadie. Cameron reassures Avery constantly, reminding her that he would do anything to protect both her and their beloved dog. Despite Cameron's loving support, Avery's obsessive fears continue to cause her significant distress, making everyday tasks and interactions challenging as she strives to keep Sadie safe from harm.

Accommodation can be subtle or overt (and extreme) and is observed in distressed and nondistressed relationships. Even if there is no obvious distress, accommodation creates a relationship "system" that fits with the OCD symptoms to perpetuate the problem. For example, accommodation might decrease a client's incentive to engage in treatment that would require a great deal of effort and change the status quo. It might also be the chief way in which loved ones have learned to show affection for the person with OCD. Not surprisingly, accommodation is related to more severe OCD symptoms and poorer long-term treatment outcome (Jacoby et al., 2021). Accordingly, reducing accommodation is an important target in treatment.

Relationship Conflict

Relationships in which one person has OCD are often characterized by interdependency, unassertiveness, and avoidant communication patterns that foster conflict. Typically, OCD symptoms and interpersonal distress influence each other (rather than one exclusively leading to the other). For example, a father's contentious relationship with his adult daughter with OCD might contribute to anxiety and uncertainty that increases the daughter's obsessional doubting. Her compulsive reassurance seeking and overly cautious behavior might also lead to frequent disagreements and conflicts with her father.

1.3 Epidemiology

OCD has a 1-year prevalence of 1.2% and a lifetime prevalence of 2.3% in the adult population (this is equivalent to about 1 in 40 adults; Ruscio et al., 2010). The disorder affects women slightly more often than men, and the age of onset, although earlier for males, is around 19 years on average.

Most individuals experience OCD symptoms for several years before receiving proper diagnosis and treatment. Factors contributing to the underrecognition of OCD include the reluctance of clients to disclose their sometimes embarrassing symptoms (see Section 4.5.12), the failure of professionals to screen for obsessions and compulsions during routine examinations (see Section 1.7.1), and difficulties with differential diagnoses (see Section 1.5).

1.4 Course and Prognosis

OCD generally runs a chronic and deteriorating course

OCD symptoms typically develop gradually. An exception is the abrupt onset sometimes observed during pregnancy or postpartum. Another putative exception is *pediatric autoimmune neuropsychiatric disorders associated with streptococcal infections* (PANDAS), which involves the abrupt onset or worsening of OCD and/or tics among children following such an infection (Swedo, 2002). The modal age of onset of OCD ranges between 6–15 years in males and 20–29 years in females. Generally, OCD has a low rate of spontaneous remission. Left untreated, the disorder runs a chronic and deteriorating course, although symptoms may wax and wane in severity over time (often dependent upon levels of psychosocial stress).

1.5 Differential Diagnoses

OCD is often confused with other disorders with seemingly similar features

In clinical practice, OCD can be difficult to differentiate from a number of problems with deceptively similar symptom patterns. Moreover, the terms "obsessive" and "compulsive" are often used indiscriminately to refer to phenomena that are not clinical obsessions and compulsions as defined by the DSM-5-TR. This section highlights key differences between the symptoms of OCD and those of several other disorders.

1.5.1 Generalized Anxiety Disorder

Anxious apprehension and repetitive thoughts are present in both OCD and *generalized anxiety disorder* (GAD). However, worries in GAD concern real-life problems (e.g., losing one's job, finances, relationships) and are typically in line with the individual's sense of self (i.e., ego-syntonic). On the other hand, obsessions in OCD often contain senseless or bizarre content that is ego-dystonic (i.e., not in line with one's sense of self). For example, rather than generally worrying about losing one's job (as in GAD), a client with OCD may be worried about sending something offensive or inappropriate in a work email by mistake that they would never normally write. Obsessions in OCD also often focus on personalized responsibility. For example, rather than generally worrying about the safety of loved ones as in GAD (e.g., "what if my husband gets in a car accident driving to work"), a client with OCD might think "what if I suddenly swerve the car when I'm driving and hit a pedestrian." Moreover, the content of worries in GAD may shift frequently, whereas the content of obsessional fears is generally stable over time.

1.5.2 Depression

OCD and depression both involve repetitive negative thoughts. However, depressive ruminations are generalized, pessimistic ideas about the self, world, or future (e.g., "no one likes me") with frequent shifts in content. Unlike obsessions, ruminations are not strongly resisted, and they do not elicit avoidance or compulsive rituals. Obsessions, on the other hand, are thoughts, ideas, and images that involve fears of specific disastrous consequences, with infrequent shifts in content.

Sometimes it can be challenging to distinguish an unwanted intrusive thought about self-harm from suicidal thoughts. Some helpful questions to ask clients include: (a) are the thoughts of harm ego-dystonic (i.e., the exact opposite of what the person wants to do; more likely OCD); (b) do the thoughts come up randomly (e.g., the person is walking down the street, and all of a sudden they have a thought of stepping in front of oncoming traffic; more likely OCD) or are they mood-congruent (i.e., do they come up when the person is feeling most depressed; more likely depression); (c) does the person feel anxious when thoughts of harm come up (more likely OCD) or do they feel a sense of comfort in thinking about ways they can kill themselves (more likely depression); (d) does the person express any intent to act on the thoughts (which would be a risk factor and also more likely indicative of depression). In summary, clients with OCD most commonly will say these thoughts come up randomly and are the exact opposite of anything they would want to do. They make clients feel anxious or fearful (e.g., wondering what these thoughts mean), and they do not want to do anything to act on them.

1.5.3 Tics and Tourette's Syndrome

Tics reduce sensory tension (vs. fear)

Both OCD and *Tourette's syndrome* (TS) involve stereotyped or repetitive movements. However, tics (as in TS) are spontaneous acts evoked by a sensory urge. They serve to reduce sensory tension rather than as an escape from obsessive fear. In contrast, compulsions in OCD are deliberate acts evoked by affective distress and the urge to reduce fear.

1.5.4 Psychotic Disorders (e.g., Schizophrenia)

Both OCD and *psychotic disorders* involve senseless and fixed thoughts and beliefs that may evoke distress. In fact, these thoughts can be conceptualized as occurring on a spectrum, with delusions seen in psychotic disorders being on the extreme end of conviction and most bizarre. For example, a client with OCD may fear that they will accidentally cheat on an exam without meaning to whereas one with psychotic delusions may be convinced that their professor is watching them through the webcam of their computer to catch them cheating on a take-home exam. Additionally, obsessions are typically inconsistent with the client's sense of self (i.e., ego-dystonic), whereas delusions, on the other hand, are integrated into a client's belief system. Furthermore, any repetitive behaviors seen in schizophrenia are in harmony with the delusional beliefs (e.g., repeatedly checking the window to confirm one is being spied on) rather than being an attempt to neutralize unwanted obsessions, and clients with schizophrenia view these behaviors as justified (rather than senseless or excessive). Schizophrenia is also accompanied by other negative symptoms of thought disorders (e.g., loosening associations) that are not present in OCD.

1.5.5 Impulsive Behavior and Habit Disorders

Excessive and repetitive behaviors might be present in both OCD and in disorders characterized by impulse control difficulties, such as pathological gambling, pathological shopping and/or buying, *body-focused repetitive behaviors* (BFRBs) including hair pulling disorder (a.k.a. trichotillomania) and skin picking disorder (a.k.a. excoriation), kleptomania, compulsive Internet use (e.g., viewing pornography, playing videogames), and sexually impulsive behaviors. For this reason, some impulse control problems (i.e., skin picking and hair pulling) are considered "obsessive-compulsive related disorders" in DSM-5-TR. However, while some BFRBs can be performed to alleviate anxiety, stress, or boredom, the repetitive behaviors in impulse control problems are typically performed to achieve a feeling of gratification (i.e., they are positively reinforced), whereas compulsive rituals in OCD are performed to escape from distress (i.e., they are negatively reinforced). Also, BFRBs can sometimes occur outside the person's awareness, whereas repetitive behaviors in OCD are typically triggered by an obsession (e.g., feeling that things are "not right"). Although individuals with impulse control problems may experience guilt, shame, and anxiety associated with their problematic behaviors and habits, their anxiety is not triggered by obsessional cues as in OCD – that is, obsessions are not present. Thus, the treatment for these impulse control problems (i.e., habit reversal training) is very different from ERP for OCD.

1.5.6 Obsessive-Compulsive Personality Disorder

Whereas OCD and *obsessive-compulsive personality disorder* (OCPD) have overlapping names, there are more differences than similarities between the two conditions. OCPD is a set of pervasive traits that involve rigidity and inflexibility, meticulousness, and sometimes impulsive anger and hostility. People with OCPD often view these traits as functional and consistent with their world view (i.e., they are ego-syntonic). On the other hand, OCD symptoms are experienced as upsetting and incongruent with the person's world view (i.e., ego-dystonic). Hence, OCD symptoms are resisted, whereas OCPD symptoms are not typically resisted because they do not cause personal distress (although others might become distressed over the person's behaviors). For example, someone with OCPD might spend excessive amounts of time ordering and arranging objects in their home but would describe these behaviors as satisfying, versus a client with OCD who would experience anxiety and distress around attempting to get their organization "just right."

1.5.7 Illness Anxiety Disorder

Persistent thoughts about illnesses and repetitive checking for reassurance can be present in both OCD and illness (or health-related) anxiety (once referred to as *hypochondriasis*). In OCD, however, clients evidence additional obsessive themes (e.g., aggression, contamination), whereas in illness anxiety disorder, clients are singly obsessed with their health. Some additional distinctions to consider:

- **Present vs. future:** Clients with illness anxiety are typically preoccupied that they have a disease currently (e.g., cancer) and perhaps the doctors have simply missed it. In contrast, obsessions in OCD are often focused on fears of getting sick in the future (e.g., contracting cancer one day due to exposure to toxic chemicals).
- **Communicable infection vs. not:** Clients with OCD are often afraid of communicable illnesses (e.g., COVID-19 or the flu), whereas clients with illness anxiety are often fearful of illnesses or diseases that may not be transmissible (e.g., heart disease).
- **Does the reassurance seeking provide relief:** Whereas clients with OCD may report temporary relief from finding out from a doctor they are healthy, clients with health anxiety often end up doubting the advice of their doctor and seeking additional opinions thinking the first doctor was simply incorrect.

1.5.8 Body Dysmorphic Disorder

Both *body dysmorphic disorder* (BDD; also an OCRD) and OCD can involve intrusive, distressing thoughts and repetitive behaviors such as checking. However, in BDD, the thoughts and behaviors are limited to preoccupation with one or more perceived flaws in physical appearance that are slight or unobservable (e.g., the symmetry of one's nose accompanied by excessive mirror checking, makeup application, social comparison, and reassurance seeking), whereas people with OCD have obsessions focused on other themes as described above. In addition, the overall level of insight into the senselessness of BDD symptoms tends to be lower than for OCD.

1.5.9 Hoarding Disorder

Hoarding is classified as its own disorder in DSM-5-TR

Once considered a symptom of OCD, *hoarding* is now its own diagnostic entity (within the OCRDs) in DSM-5-TR. The primary symptoms are excessive acquisition of large quantities of objects (e.g., old newspapers and clothes) that cover the living areas of the home and the inability or unwillingness to discard these objects even though they might impede activities such as cooking, cleaning, moving through the house, and sleeping. Although the collection of objects (and failure to discard them) can appear "compulsive" (and might sometimes be part of OCD-related rituals; e.g., needing to know and remember things, fear of mistakenly discarding something important, or not wanting to touch items perceived to be contaminated resulting in clutter), difficulty discarding is typically not motivated by obsessional fear as in OCD, but rather by reasons such as aesthetics (thinking an item is beautiful), utility (possibly needing the item later), not wanting to waste the item, emotional and sentimental attachment, control and ownership over the item, etc. In other words, the person with hoarding disorder often derives pleasure from saving things. Typically, excessive acquisition of items (i.e., to the extent that someone is unable to use rooms in their home) would indicate a diagnosis of hoarding (vs. one of OCD).

1.6 Comorbidity Rates

Comorbidity is common in OCD

The most frequently co-occurring diagnoses among people with OCD are depressive and anxiety disorders. First, about 50% of people with OCD have experienced at least one major depressive episode (or dysthymia) in their lives. When comorbid depression is present, OCD typically pre-dates the depressive symptoms, suggesting that depressive symptoms usually occur in response to the distress and functional impairment associated with OCD (rather than as a precursor). Depressive symptoms also seem to be more strongly related to the severity of obsessions than to compulsions. Commonly co-occurring anxiety disorders include GAD, panic disorder, and social anxiety disorder, with rates ranging from 30% to 45% (Hirschtritt et al., 2017). Less frequently, individuals with OCD have comorbid eating disorders, tic disorders (e.g., Tourette's syndrome), and impulse control disorders. Studies generally agree that personality disorders belonging to the anxious cluster (e.g., obsessive-compulsive, avoidant) more commonly co-occur with OCD than those of other clusters (Hirschtritt et al., 2017). Considerations for treatment in the context of these comorbidities are discussed in Section 3.4.10.

1.7 Diagnostic Procedures and Documentation

This section reviews the empirically established structured and semistructured diagnostic interviews and self-report measures for assessing the presence and severity of OCD symptoms, as well as for documenting changes in these symptoms during a course of psychological treatment.

1.7.1 Screening

The Obsessive-Compulsive Inventory–4 is a brief four-item screener for OCD

The *Obsessive-Compulsive Inventory-4* (OCI-4; Abramovitch et al., 2021) is a four-item self-report measure designed to screen for likely OCD symptoms. It assesses common dimensions of OCD, including washing, checking, obsessional thoughts, and the need for order and symmetry. Each item is rated on a Likert scale, providing a quick evaluation of the severity of OCD-related symptoms. A score of 3 or above suggests the need for further assessment to determine whether a clinical diagnosis of OCD is appropriate. The OCI-4 is freely available on the Internet at https://static1.squarespace.com/static/56d5ca187da24ffed7378b40/t/61de37dfa41a455c016192b0/1641953248179/OCI4+FORM.pdf.

1.7.2 Structured Diagnostic Interviews

Several structured diagnostic interviews that are based on DSM-5-TR criteria can be used to confirm the diagnosis of OCD: the *Anxiety and Related Disorders Interview Schedule for DSM-5* (ADIS-5; Brown & Barlow, 2014), the *Structured Clinical Interview for DSM-5* (SCID; First et al., 2015), the *Diagnostic Interview for Anxiety Mood and OCD-Related Neuropsychiatric Disorders* (DIAMOND; Tolin et al., 2018), and the *Mini International Neuropsychiatric Interview* (MINI; Sheehan et al., 1998). Each of these instruments possess good reliability and validity. The DIAMOND is freely available over the Internet (https://giving.hartfordhospital.org/tolin-diamond-training-video/), and the other measures are available for purchase (ADIS: Oxford University Press; SCID: American Psychiatric Association; MINI: https://harmresearch.org/mini-international-neuropsychiatric-interview-mini/).

1.7.3 Semistructured Symptom Interviews

OCD is unique among the psychological disorders in that the form and content of its symptoms can vary widely from one person to the next. In fact, two individuals with OCD might present with completely nonoverlapping symptoms. Such heterogeneity necessitates a thorough assessment of the *topography* of the individual's symptoms: what types of obsessions and compulsions are present, and how severe are these symptoms?

Yale-Brown Obsessive Compulsive Scale (Y-BOCS)

The Y-BOCS is a measure of OCD symptom severity

The *Yale-Brown Obsessive Compulsive Scale* (Y-BOCS; Goodman, Price, Rasmussen, Mazure, Delgado, et al., 1989; Goodman, Price, Rasmussen, Mazure, Fleischmann, et al., 1989), which includes a symptom checklist and a severity rating scale, is ideal for addressing these questions. Between 30 and 60 minutes might be required to administer this semistructured interview. The first part of the symptom checklist provides definitions and examples of obsessions and compulsions that the clinician reads to the client. Next, the clinician reviews a comprehensive list of over 50 common obsessions and compulsions, and asks the client whether each symptom is currently present or has occurred in the past. Finally, the most prominent obsessions, compulsions, and OCD-related avoidance behaviors are listed. A benefit of this checklist is it can encourage clients who would be reluctant to spontaneously share unacceptable thoughts (e.g., about violence or sex) to come forward with these symptoms once prompted about them on the checklist (i.e., normalizing these obsessional thoughts as common).

One limitation of the Y-BOCS symptom checklist is that it assesses obsessions and compulsions according to *form* rather than *function*. It is therefore up to the clinician to inquire about the relationship between obsessions and compulsions (i.e., which obsessional thoughts evoke which rituals). A second limitation is that the checklist inadequately assesses the breadth of mental rituals. Thus, the clinician must probe in a less structured way for the presence of these covert symptoms. The assessment of mental rituals is discussed further in Section 4.1.1. Finally, there are several obsessions and compulsions on the checklist that could be tied to OCD or may be related to another disorder; however, additional guidance about differential diagnosis is not given. For example, "fear of doing something else embarrassing" could be an obsession as seen in OCD (e.g., blurting out gibberish in a meeting which the individual would probably never actually do), or it could be characteristic of social anxiety. Thus, clinicians should conduct a careful assessment to ensure that endorsed items are indeed OCD.

The Y-BOCS severity scale includes 10 items to assess the following five parameters of obsessions (items 1–5) and compulsions (items 6–10): (a) time, (b) interference, (c) distress, (d) efforts to resist, and (e) perceived control. Each item is rated on a scale from 0 to 4, and the item scores are summed to produce a total score ranging from 0 (*no symptoms*) to 40 (*extreme*). Table 1 shows the clinical breakdown of scores on the Y-BOCS severity scale. The measure has acceptable reliability, validity, and sensitivity to change. An advantage of the Y-BOCS is that it assesses OCD symptom severity independent of symptom content. However, a drawback of this approach, as mentioned above with the checklist, is that the clinician must be cautious to avoid rating the symptoms of other problems (e.g., GAD, impulse control problems) as obsessions or compulsions. Another limitation is that avoidance is not directly assessed by the Y-BOCS severity items (there is an adjunct avoidance item, but it is not included in the total score). Raters can, however, use the interference items to capture the effects of avoidance.

Table 1
Clinical Breakdown of Scores on the Y-BOCS Severity Scale (based on Storch et al., 2015)

Y-BOCS score	Clinical severity
0–7	Subclinical
8–13	Mild
14–25	Moderate
26–34	Moderate to severe
35–40	Severe

Note. Y-BOCS = Yale-Brown Obsessive Compulsive Scale.

Brown Assessment of Beliefs Scale

The BABS is a measure of insight in OCD

Since poor insight has been linked to attenuated treatment outcome, the assessment of OCD should include determination of the extent to which the client perceives their obsessions and compulsions as senselessness and excessive. The *Brown Assessment of Beliefs Scale* (BABS; Eisen et al., 1998) is a semistructured interview that contains seven items and assesses insight as a continuous variable. The client first identifies one or two current obsessional fears (e.g., "If I touch dirty laundry without washing my hands, I will become sick"). Next, individual items assess (a) conviction in this belief, (b) perceptions of how others view this belief, (c) explanation for why others hold a different view, (d) willingness to challenge the belief, (e) attempts to disprove the belief, (f) insight into the senselessness of the belief, and (g) ideas or delusions of reference. Each item is rated on a scale from 0 to 4, and the first six items are summed to obtain a total score of 0 to 24 (higher scores indicate poorer insight). The seventh item is not included in the total score. The BABS has good reliability, validity, and sensitivity to change. Of note, the Y-BOCS also has a single adjunct item that assesses insight, but that does not factor into the total score.

1.7.4 Self-Report Inventories

Self-report inventories are used to gather additional severity data

Psychometrically validated self-report questionnaires can be used to supplement the clinical interviews described above. Such questionnaires are easily administered, carefully worded, and have well-established norms. Accordingly, they are best used to corroborate information obtained from clinical interviewing and to monitor symptom severity during treatment.

Dimensional Obsessive-Compulsive Scale

The DOCS is a brief measure of OCD severity

The *Dimensional Obsessive-Compulsive Scale* (DOCS) is a 20-item measure that assesses the severity of the four most consistently replicated OCD symptom dimensions, which correspond to the measure's four subscales: (a) contamination, (b) responsibility for harm and mistakes, (c) symmetry/ordering/incompleteness, and (d) unacceptable/taboo obsessions. Each subscale begins with a description of the symptom dimension, along with examples of representative obsessions and rituals. The examples clarify the form and function of each dimension's fundamental obsessional fears, compulsive rituals, and avoidance behaviors. Each subscale contains five items (rated 0 to 4) to assess the following parameters of severity: (a) time occupied by obsessions and rituals, (b) avoidance behavior, (c) associated distress, (d) functional interference, and (e) difficulty disregarding the obsessions and refraining from the compulsions. Scores for each subscale (symptom dimension) range from 0 to 20. The DOCS subscales have excellent reliability, validity, and sensitivity to treatment effects (Abramowitz et al., 2010). Total scores of at least 18 or 21 can help distinguish people with OCD from those with no disorder or an anxiety disorder, respectively. The DOCS is freely available on the Internet (https://docs.web.unc.edu/).

Measures of General Functioning

The WSAS captures OCD-related functional impairment

The *Work and Social Adjustment Scale* (WSAS; Mundt et al. 2002) is a 5-item self-report scale assessing interference in work, home management, social leisure activities, private leisure activities, and close relationships, each rated on a scale from 0 (*not at all impaired*) to 8 (*very severely impaired*). Clients can be instructed to complete this measure specifically regarding impairment due to their OCD. Thus, scores on each individual item can be informative, and items can also be summed for a global measure of impairment ranging from 0 to 40, with higher scores indicating greater impairment.

1.7.5 Documenting Changes in Symptom Levels

Assessing OCD symptoms throughout treatment

Continual assessment of OCD and related symptoms throughout the course of psychological treatment assists the clinician in evaluating treatment response. It is not enough to simply assume that "he seems to be less obsessed," or "it looks like she has cut down on her compulsions," or even for the client to report that they now "feel better." We recommend periodic assessment and comparison with baseline symptom levels (e.g., monthly) using psychometrically validated self-report and interview measures to clarify objectively in what ways treatment has been helpful and what work remains to be done.

2

Theories and Models

A number of theories have been proposed to explain the development and clinical picture of OCD. This chapter reviews the most well-studied theoretical models, with an emphasis on the cognitive-behavioral perspective which forms the basis of the treatment program described in Chapter 4.

2.1 Biological Theories

2.1.1 Neurotransmitter Theories

Few data suggest that problems with neurotransmitters mediate OCD symptoms

Biological models of OCD can be categorized into neurotransmitter and neuroanatomical theories. Prevailing *neurotransmitter theories* propose that abnormalities in the serotonin system, particularly the hypersensitivity of postsynaptic serotonergic receptors, underlie OCD symptoms. This *serotonin hypothesis* was proposed following observations that serotonergic medication, but not other kinds of antidepressants, were effective in reducing OCD symptoms. However, results from numerous studies that have directly examined the serotonin system and its relationship to OCD do not support this hypothesis. Whereas the preferential response of OCD to serotonergic medication is often championed as supporting the serotonin hypothesis, this argument is of little value since the hypothesis was derived from this treatment outcome result. Abnormalities in the dopamine system, which is involved in reward processing and motor functions, and the glutamate system, an excitatory neurotransmitter in the brain, have also been proposed as contributing to OCD. However, to date there are limited data to suggest that problems with these neurotransmitter functioning mediate OCD symptoms.

2.1.2 Neuroanatomical Theories

Predominant *neuroanatomical models* of OCD propose that obsessions and compulsions arise from structural and functional abnormalities in particular areas of the brain, specifically the orbitofrontal-subcortical circuits. These circuits are thought to connect regions of the brain involved in processing information with those involved in the initiation of certain behavioral responses, and their overactivity is thought to lead to OCD. Neuroanatomical models have been derived from imaging studies in which activity levels in specific parts of the brain are compared between clients with OCD and healthy controls without OCD. For example, functional magnetic resonance imaging (fMRI) studies have consistently found increased activation in the orbitofrontal cortex (OFC) among clients with OCD as compared with controls.

Although thought-provoking, imaging studies are cross-sectional and correlational, and therefore cannot address hypotheses about cause, such as whether OCD arises from apparent dysfunctions in the brain or whether the observed alterations in brain function represent normally functioning brain systems that are simply affected by the presence of chronic obsessional anxiety; thus, the direction of causality remains unclear. Moreover, to date there is no biological (i.e., neurochemical, neuroanatomical, or genetic) test for OCD.

2.2 Psychological Theories

2.2.1 Learning Theory

Early learning (conditioning) models explain some aspects of OCD (but not others)

Early learning (conditioning) models of OCD were drawn from Mowrer's (1960) two-factor theory which proposes that pathological fear is acquired by classical conditioning and maintained by operant conditioning. For example, an obsessional fear of cemeteries is thought to arise from an experience during which anxiety becomes associated with such places. This fear is then maintained by behaviors that prevent the natural extinction of the fear, such as avoidance of cemeteries and compulsive praying. Avoidance and rituals are negatively reinforced by the immediate (albeit temporary) reduction in discomfort that they engender. Thus, such behaviors develop into strong habits.

Research supports some aspects of the learning theory, but not others. For example, obsessional stimuli indeed *evoke* anxiety, and compulsive rituals do bring about an immediate *reduction* in anxiety and distress. However, traumatic conditioning experiences do not appear to be necessary for the development of obsessions. Contemporary cognitive-behavioral models (as described in Section 2.2.3) were subsequently formulated to explain the development of obsessional fear.

2.2.2 Cognitive Deficit Models

Cognitive deficit models have two key limitations

Because people with OCD sometimes demonstrate the appearance of reduced performance on cognitive tasks such as executive functioning, cognitive inhibition, and some forms of memory, some theorists have proposed that OCD is characterized by deficits in neuropsychological and information-processing functioning. However, such impairment, if present at all, tends to be mild and of little clinical importance (Abramovitch et al., 2013). Moreover, these minor deficits could result from the effects of obsessional anxiety and fear (as opposed to the other way around). *Cognitive deficit models* have two key limitations. First, they do not account for the heterogeneity of OCD symptoms (e.g., why some individuals have contamination obsessions and others have obsessions about making mistakes). Second, because mild cognitive deficits are present in many psychological disorders (e.g., panic disorder, bulimia nervosa), these models fail to explain why such deficits give rise to OCD instead of a different disorder. Thus, if cognitive deficits play a causal role in OCD at all, they most likely represent a nonspecific vulnerability factor. Additionally, an alternative explanation is the fact that people with OCD have reduced *confidence* in their memory and other cognitive functions (e.g., doubting whether one turned off the stove, leading to checking behaviors that undermine one's memory confidence even further) which could contribute to these cognitive deficits.

2.2.3 Contemporary Cognitive-Behavioral Models

Contemporary cognitive-behavioral models of OCD form the basis for ERP

Cognitive-behavioral approaches to OCD, which serve as the basis for the treatment program described in this book, begin with the well-established finding that intrusive thoughts (i.e., negative thoughts, images, and doubts that intrude into consciousness) are normal experiences for just about everyone from time to time. Sometimes triggered by external stimuli (e.g., thoughts of harm that are triggered by the sight of a kitchen knife), such intrusions usually reflect themes that are of importance to the person (e.g., health and safety, religion and morality, etc.).

The cognitive-behavioral model proposes that the mistaken appraisal of these normal intrusions as personally significant and threatening (i.e., an alarm or "call to action") is what leads the intrusions to develop into highly distressing and time-consuming obsessional preoccupations. For example, consider the unwanted thought of verbally abusing a beloved older family member. Most people would consider such an intrusion as meaningless or harmless (e.g., "mental noise"). However, according to the cognitive-behavioral model, such an intrusion would develop into a clinical obsession if the person were to attach to it a high degree of importance, leading to an escalation in negative emotion and doubt; for example, "Thinking about verbally abusing Grand-pop means I'm a terrible person who must be extra careful to make sure I don't do something terrible." Such appraisals evoke distress, uncertainty, and motivate the person to try to (a) control, suppress, or neutralize the unwanted thought (e.g., by praying or replacing it with a "safe" thought); (b) attempt to prevent any harmful events associated with the intrusion (e.g., by avoiding older people), or (c) gain certainty regarding any possible feared consequences (e.g., seeking reassurance).

Compulsive rituals are conceptualized as efforts to control or reduce obsessional distress and anxiety, remove unwanted intrusions, and gain certainty that feared consequences will not occur. However, rituals are counterproductive for a number of reasons. First, because they are sometimes temporarily "effective" in providing the desired reduction in distress, these strategies are negatively reinforced and frequently evolve into time-consuming patterns that impair functioning and quality of life. Second, because they provide an immediate (albeit fleeting) escape from anxiety and doubt, rituals prevent the person from learning that thoughts, anxiety, and uncertainty are manageable. Third, rituals prevent the person from learning that obsessional distress eventually abates naturally even without performing rituals. Fourth, rituals lead to an increase in the frequency of obsessions by serving as reminders of obsessional intrusions, thereby triggering the person's intense preoccupation with the very thought they are trying to suppress. For example, compulsively checking the stove can trigger intrusions about house fires. Attempts at distracting oneself from unwanted intrusions may paradoxically increase the frequency of intrusions, possibly because the distractors become reminders (retrieval cues) of the intrusions. Finally, performing rituals preserves dysfunctional beliefs and misinterpretations of obsessional thoughts. That is, when feared consequences do not occur after performance of a ritual, the person (erroneously) attributes this to the ritual that was performed, rather than (correctly) to the innocuousness of the intrusion.

Brief summary of the cognitive-behavioral approach to OCD

To summarize, when a person appraises an otherwise normally occurring mental intrusion as threatening and personally significant, they become distressed and attempt to control or remove the intrusion, reduce uncertainty, and prevent the feared consequences. This paradoxically increases the frequency of intrusions. Thus, the intrusions escalate into persistent and distressing clinical obsessions to which the person becomes exquisitely sensitive. Because the obsessional thought is experienced as distressing, it evokes urges to perform some response – overt or covert – to neutralize the distress and bring about assurance of safety. Compulsions maintain the intrusions and prevent the self-correction of mistaken (catastrophic) appraisals and the belief that one cannot manage with the associated anxiety and uncertainty. Table 2 summarizes the various factors that maintain OCD symptoms.

Misinterpretations of one's thoughts might include any appraisal of the intrusive thought as personally significant or threatening. An example is the belief that thinking about bad behavior is morally equivalent to performing the corresponding behavior (e.g., "Thinking about cheating is as bad as actually cheating"). An international group of researchers interested in the cognitive basis of OCD, the Obsessive Compulsive Cognitions Working Group (OCCWG; Frost & Steketee, 2002) identified three domains of *core beliefs* thought to underlie the development of obsessions from normal intrusive thoughts. These are summarized in Table 3. Figure 1 graphically depicts the contemporary cognitive-behavioral conceptual model. It is important to point out that, like the other models, questions remain regarding the cognitive-behavioral approach. Although research consistently supports the tenants of this model in general, cognitive and behavioral factors do not account completely for OCD symptoms. Thus, there are likely other factors involved in the development and maintenance of the problem.

Table 2
Summary of Maintenance Processes in OCD

Maintenance process	Description
Selective attention	Hypervigilance for threat cues enhances the detection of obsessional stimuli.
Physiological factors	The fight-or-flight response is a normal response to perceived threat. Emotional reasoning reaffirms mistaken beliefs that lead to feeling anxious.
Anxiety-reduction behaviors	Overt and covert rituals, reassurance seeking, and neutralizing strategies are reinforced by the immediate reduction in distress they engender. In the long-term, these strategies prevent disconfirmation of mistaken beliefs, because of how their outcomes are incorrectly interpreted.
Passive avoidance	Avoidance produces temporary anxiety reduction but prevents disconfirmation of overestimates of risk, because the person never has the opportunity to find out that the danger is unlikely.
Concealment of obsessions	Hiding obsessions from others prevents disconfirmation of mistaken beliefs about the normalcy of intrusive thoughts.
Attempted thought control	Attempts to control or suppress unwanted thoughts lead to an increase in unwanted thoughts. Misappraisal of thought control failure leads to further distress.
Experiential avoidance	The tendency to evade or escape unpleasant thoughts, feelings, or body sensations, even when doing so interferes with one's functioning (i.e., psychological inflexibility).

Table 3
Domains of Pathogenic Beliefs in OCD

Belief	Description
Inflated responsibility and overestimation of threat	Belief that one has the power to cause and/or the duty to prevent negative outcomes featured in intrusive thoughts. Belief that negative events associated with intrusive thoughts are likely and would be insufferable.
Exaggeration of the importance of thoughts and need to control thoughts	Belief that the mere presence of a thought indicates that the thought is significant. Belief that complete control over one's thoughts is both necessary and possible.
Perfectionism and intolerance of uncertainty	Belief that mistakes and imperfection are intolerable. Belief that it is necessary and possible to be 100% certain that negative outcomes will not occur.

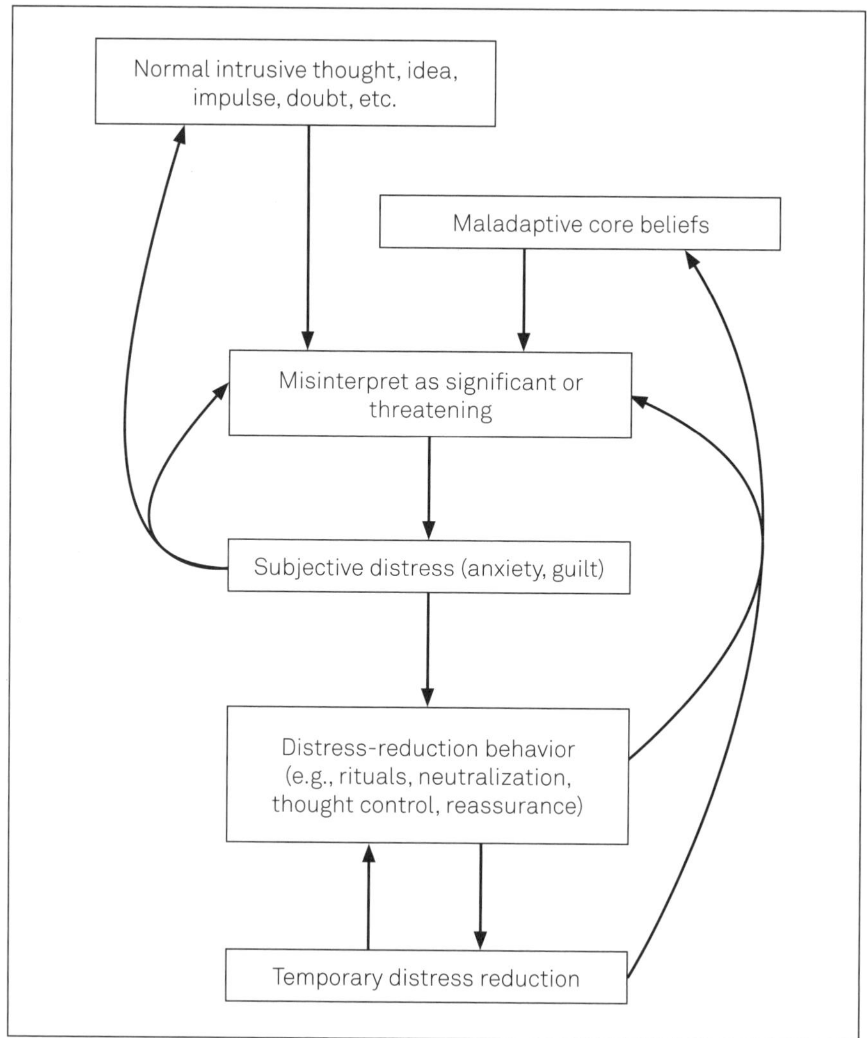

Figure 1
Cognitive-behavioral conceptual model of OCD.

Implications of the Cognitive-Behavioral Model

Normalizing Effects

The cognitive-behavioral approach assumes no brain dysfunctions

The cognitive-behavioral approach provides a logically and empirically consistent account of OCD symptoms that assumes the presence of intact learning (conditioning) processes and normally functioning (albeit maladaptive) cognitive processes. There is no appeal to chemical imbalances or broken brain parts to explain OCD symptoms. Even the maladaptive beliefs and assumptions that lead to obsessions are viewed as *cognitive biases* rather than *disease processes*. Furthermore, avoidance and compulsive rituals to reduce perceived threat and uncertainty would be considered adaptive if danger were indeed present. However, obsessive fears are exaggerated, and therefore, avoidance and safety-seeking rituals are not only unnecessary, but maladaptive, since they perpetuate a vicious cycle of intrusion -> misappraisal -> anxiety, that causes a reduction in quality of life.

Vulnerability to OCD

The distal cause of OCD is unknown, but the problem's etiology probably involves interactions among (as yet not well-understood) biological, genetic, and environmental variables. Cognitive-behavioral models propose that certain experiences lead people to develop core beliefs that underlie OCD. For example, an obsession could develop in someone who was taught high moral standards and expected to obey rigid and extreme codes of conduct where the threat of punishment for disobedience was constantly present (e.g., as in certain strict religious doctrines). However, empirical evidence supporting the role of these kinds of experiences in the etiology of OCD is equivocal, and many clients with OCD do not describe such experiences in their past.

For those who develop OCD, however, clinical experience does suggest that OCD latches onto the things they care most about (i.e., their values). Accordingly, clients with concerns about germs or contamination tend to be the ones who care the most about health and cleanliness, those with unacceptable taboo thoughts about violence tend to be the gentlest and most caring people, those with obsessions about symmetry and exactness tend to be those who are most organized, etc. Studies conducted around the world show that certain presentations of OCD are elevated depending on the cultural values of the region (e.g., elevated levels of scrupulosity in religious cultures) providing empirical support for this idea (e.g., Hunt, 2020).

Treatment Implications of the Model

ERP should target maladaptive beliefs and distress-reduction behaviors

The cognitive-behavioral model identifies specific targets for reducing OCD symptoms. In particular, effective treatment must help clients (a) correct maladaptive beliefs and appraisals that lead to obsessional fear and (b) decrease avoidance and rituals that prevent the self-correction of maladaptive beliefs. In short, the task of ERP is to foster a healthier perspective toward obsessional stimuli (situations, stimuli, thoughts, and internal sensations) as acceptable, safe, and manageable, and therefore not demanding the need to reduce anxiety or gain certainty about feared consequences. Clients must come to understand their problem not in terms of the risk of feared consequences, but in terms of how they are relating to stimuli that pose a low risk to them and are indeed a universal human experience. Those with aggressive obsessions must view their problem as that of lending too much significance to meaningless intrusive thoughts (instead of how they are going to achieve the ultimate guarantee that feared consequences will not occur). Clients with washing rituals must see their problem not as needing a sure-fire way to prevent illness, but as the need to change how they evaluate and respond to situations that realistically pose a low risk of illness. The treatment procedures outlined in Chapter 4 are derived from the learning and cognitive-behavioral models of OCD to address these targets.

3

Diagnosis and Treatment Indications

This chapter provides a framework for conducting a diagnostic assessment and providing consultation regarding the treatment of OCD. The cognitive-behavioral model and its treatment implications (see Chapter 2) determine how information about the client's symptoms is assessed and conceptualized. The initial consultation provides an excellent opportunity to initiate rapport building and begin socializing the client to the treatment approach.

3.1 Form Versus Function

The cognitive-behavioral model emphasizes functional aspects of OCD symptoms

Whereas the diagnostic criteria for OCD emphasize descriptions of obsessions and compulsions, the cognitive-behavioral model emphasizes the *functional* aspects of these phenomena. From this perspective, the essential features of OCD are anxiety-evoking obsessional thoughts and anxiety-reducing strategies such as rituals and avoidance. It is the person's maladaptive beliefs and appraisals of obsessional stimuli which give rise to obsessional fear. Thus, it is important to assess how the client gives meaning to obsessional stimuli. Whereas *compulsiveness* and repetition might be the most outwardly observable signs of OCD, clients may deploy a variety of escape and avoidance behaviors in response to obsessional distress, and only some of these behaviors are repetitive or "compulsive". Table 4 shows the array of *safety behaviors* that might be observed in OCD. It is also important to assess how the client's safety behaviors are related to obsessional stimuli and dysfunctional thinking patterns.

Research indicates the presence of different OCD symptom dimensions involving specific types of obsessions and rituals or safety behaviors (McKay et al., 2004). Table 5 shows the most commonly identified OCD symptom dimensions.

Table 4
Types of Safety Behaviors Observed in OCD

Type	Examples
Passive avoidance	Avoidance of situations and stimuli (e.g., driving, being the last one to leave the house, toilets, the number 666); procrastination of activities that will trigger distress and/or compulsions
Compulsive rituals	Hand washing, checking, seeking reassurance, repeating routine activities
Covert neutralizing	Mental rituals (e.g., repeating prayers, "good" words, or "safe" phrases; mental reviewing when one previously left the house and locked the door; self-reassurance that feared outcomes won't occur); brief mental acts (e.g., canceling out a "bad" thought with a "good" thought), thought suppression, mental distraction
Brief or subtle mini rituals	Use of wipes or paper towels as a barrier when touching contaminated surfaces, quick checks of appliances, scrutinizing others' behavior or facial expressions

Table 5
Common OCD symptom presentations

Symptom presentation	Commonly observed symptoms
Contamination	Obsessions concerning contamination from dirt, germs, body secretions, household items, poisonous materials; washing and cleaning rituals, avoidance
Harm	Obsessions concerning responsibility for injury or harm to others; compulsive checking, seeking reassurance, repeating activities to prevent disasters
Incompleteness	Obsessions concerning order, asymmetry, imbalance (perhaps the fear that discomfort will persist indefinitely); compulsive arranging, ordering, repeating; can occur with or without magical thinking (i.e., the belief that completing these rituals protects oneself or loved ones from harm)
Unacceptable thoughts	Obsessional thoughts, impulses, images of sex, sacrilege, and violence; mental rituals, neutralizing, seeking reassurance, avoidance

3.2 The Diagnostic Assessment

How to conduct a diagnostic assessment for OCD

The *diagnostic interview* begins with the client providing a general description of their problem, and the effects on functioning and quality of life, as well as the reasons for seeking help. Be sure to ascertain the functional relationship between obsessions and rituals as described in Section 3.1. Also, assess the onset and historical course of the problem; social, developmental, and medical history; cultural and familial factors that might impact OCD; personal and family history of psychiatric treatment; substance use patterns (i.e., alcohol, marijuana, tobacco, and other recreational drugs); and exercise and sleep habits. In addition, assess the treatment history (particularly treatment for OCD) as this may influence your current recommendations. Once this information has been obtained, use the Y-BOCS, BABS, and DOCS to gather additional severity data.

Three additional self-report instruments, the *Obsessional Beliefs Questionnaire* (OBQ), *Interpretations of Intrusions Inventory* (III; Obsessive Compulsive Cognitions Working Group, 2005), and the *Acceptance and Action Questionnaire for OCD* (AAQ-OCD; Jacoby et al., 2018) can be administered to assess OCD-related dysfunctional beliefs and experiential avoidance (i.e., those described in Table 3). The OBQ and III are reprinted in the edited volume by Frost and Steketee (2002) on cognitive aspects of OCD, and the AAQ-OCD can be found online (http://www.jabramowitz.com/ocd-aaq.html).

Clinical Pearl

When Clients Report Obsessions or Compulsions in Isolation

Whereas the majority of clients with OCD readily describe obsessional fears and compulsive rituals, some present with complaints of "pure obsessions" or "compulsions without obsessions." When assessing such clients, keep in mind that more than 90% of people with OCD report both obsessions and compulsions. Thus, you might need to conduct a more in-depth functional analysis. For individuals reporting only obsessions, this means inquiring about the use of any anxiety-reduction strategies (mental rituals or subtle behavioral or cognitive neutralizing or avoidance) that might be functioning to maintain obsessional fear. Most clients do not recognize subtle safety behaviors as OCD symptoms, or might confuse mental rituals and obsessions, but these mental rituals maintain obsessional fear just as surely as overt rituals. If these phenomena are not present, perhaps the "obsessions" are not intrusive or anxiety-evoking and therefore are not indicative of OCD (e.g., perhaps they are depressive ruminations or worries as in GAD).

When clients describe compulsive behaviors but fail to define obsessional fear, inquire about what triggers these behaviors. Sometimes clients will lead by describing problematic behaviors like checking the stove is turned off, for example, and only after probing will share that these behaviors are driven by the fear of their home burning down. If compulsions are not evoked by specific intrusive or distressing thoughts or situations as described in Chapter 1, however, OCD might not be the correct diagnosis. Perhaps an impulse-control (e.g., trichotillomania) or tic disorder is present. You can use the Y-BOCS checklist, self-report questionnaires, and detailed inquiry regarding the functional aspects of reported symptoms to rule in or rule out the diagnosis of OCD.

3.3 Identifying the Appropriate Treatment

Practice guidelines for the treatment of OCD (which can be found online at https://iocdf.org/ocd-treatment-guide/) identify two first-line treatments for OCD: CBT involving ERP and *pharmacotherapy* involving serotonin reuptake inhibitor (SRI) medication. This section briefly describes these treatments and their advantages and disadvantages.

There are two first-line treatments for OCD

Medication for OCD

Table 6 displays the brand names, generic names, and therapeutic doses of medications studied using randomized controlled trials for OCD. These agents are thought to reduce OCD by increasing the concentration of serotonin. On average, SRIs produce a 20–40% improvement in OCD symptoms over a 12-week period. There are various advantages and disadvantages to using SRI medication for treating OCD, and these are listed in the following sections:

Table 6
Medications With Demonstrated Efficacy for Treating OCD

Brand name	Generic name	Therapeutic dose
Anafranil	Clomipramine	At least 250 mg/day
Zoloft	Sertraline	At least 200 mg/day
Prozac	Fluoxetine	60–80 mg/day
Luvox	Fluvoxamine	200–300 mg/day
Paxil	Paroxetine	At least 60 mg/day
Celexa	Citalopram	At least 60 mg/day
Lexapro	Escitalopram	At least 20 mg/day

Note. For each of these, at least one double-blind randomized controlled trial exists in which the medication was more effective than a placebo.

Advantages of Medication

- Generally safe and easy to use
- Clinically effective: 20–40% symptom reduction on average for most people with OCD

Disadvantages of Medication

- Limited improvement rates
- A substantial minority of clients show little or no response
- Possibility of side effects
- Must be used continuously to sustain improvement

Cognitive-Behavior Therapy for OCD

Exposure and response prevention are the centerpiece of CBT

CBT is a multicomponent approach based on an understanding of how OCD symptoms are *maintained* (rather than its putative *causes*). The psychoeducational component entails socializing the client to the cognitive-behavioral model and providing an explanation of, and rationale for, the individual treatment techniques. Cognitive techniques for OCD involve rational discussion to help the client identify and correct mistaken beliefs that underlie obsessional fears, avoidance, and safety-seeking behaviors. ACT techniques may be used to help clients learn and practice more adaptive ways to relate to their obsessional anxiety while still pursing what they value in life.

Exposure and response prevention are the centerpiece of CBT for OCD. *Exposure* entails engaging with situations and thoughts that evoke obsessive fear. This is often accompanied by imagining the feared consequences of exposure. For example, an individual who fears contamination and sickness from garbage cans would practice touching garbage cans and then imagine being contaminated with germs and coming down with an illness. The procedure involves the client remaining in the feared situation, without performing compulsive rituals or safety behaviors, and observing that feared consequences are unlikely and that they can manage the associated distress and uncertainty evoked during the exposure. Thus, the *response prevention* component of ERP entails refraining from any behaviors (behavioral and mental rituals, subtle avoidance, and reassurance seeking) that serve to reduce obsessional anxiety or terminate exposure. For example, the client described above would refrain from cleaning rituals after touching garbage cans.

ERP facilitates extinction of obsessional fear by helping the client develop new learning that obsessional cues are generally safe and manageable. This new learning competes with existing fear-based associations. When ERP is carried out in certain ways that we illustrate in Chapter 4, the new learning inhibits the older fear-based associations (i.e., maximizing inhibitory learning), and the client recognizes that obsessional fears are excessive and that rituals are not necessary to prevent disasters or reduce distress.

As with medication treatment, there are advantages and disadvantages to ERP. These are as follows:

Advantages of ERP

- Clinically effective: 60%–70% symptom reduction on average
- Treatment is fairly brief (usually 15 to 20 sessions)
- Long-term maintenance of treatment gains is common

Disadvantages of ERP

- Client must work hard to achieve improvement and prevent relapse
- Involves purposely evoking anxiety during exposure
- Not widely available due to a relative lack of well-trained clinicians

3.4 Factors That Influence Treatment Decisions

This section considers factors that influence clinical decisions regarding which type of treatment to recommend for a particular client with OCD. Clients don't necessarily need to choose between medications vs. ERP and may pursue both treatment approaches simultaneously. However, the below guidelines are a helpful starting place for making these decisions.

Several important client factors may influence decisions about treatment

3.4.1 Age

CBT involving ERP is the first-line treatment for all age groups with OCD. Compared with young and middle-aged adults, children and older persons tend to have more difficulty with adherence to medication. Older persons are more vulnerable to drug side effects, due to reduced metabolic rate and possible interactions with other medicines. Family accommodation conflict can interfere with ERP in children. Older persons may also be less cognitively flexible, which could contraindicate ERP.

3.4.2 Sex and Gender

Sex and gender do not appear to influence the outcome of ERP. However, some clients feel more comfortable with a therapist of the same sex or gender, especially if sexual or contamination concerns are present (e.g., fears of touching one's genitals). The sex and gender of the therapist would also need to be taken into account if exposures are being done with clients in public restrooms (e.g., locating single stall or all gender bathrooms).

3.4.3 Ethnic and Racial Background

Some members of racial and ethnic minority groups are uncomfortable receiving psychological treatments, and prefer pharmacotherapy over ERP, as medication carries less stigma. Such individuals might be less willing to report embarrassing symptoms to the therapist or perform exposure tasks in public settings. In some cases, working with a therapist who identifies as a member of the same racial or ethnic group can help alleviate this problem. Despite these issues, there is no evidence that one's ethnic or racial background interferes with the ability to achieve clinically significant improvement with ERP (Williams et al., 1998).

3.4.4 Educational Level and Cognitive Impairments

Successful ERP requires that the client grasp a theoretical model of OCD and a rationale for treatment. Some handouts might be modified and simplified for clients with limited formal education to achieve a manageable reading level. Clients must also be able to implement challenging treatment procedures on their own and consolidate information learned during exposure exercises. These tasks may be difficult for individuals who are very concrete in their thinking. Medication might be recommended for developmentally disabled and cognitively impaired clients.

3.4.5 Client Preference

Client preference should be considered

Preference for a particular treatment modality should be considered. Reviewing the advantages and disadvantages of each approach allows the client to make an informed decision about which therapy they would prefer to receive. Greater adherence to either treatment (especially ERP) can be expected from clients who agree willingly to a particular plan, as opposed to those situations in which they are not given a choice between options, or treatment is forced on them. For example, because ERP involves a substantial amount of between session work, clients undergoing ERP should be committed to this approach.

3.4.6 Clinical Presentation

ERP targets obsessions and compulsions. Thus, if such symptoms are not primary complaints, it is not recommended. Because this type of treatment requires a substantial commitment, we recommend that it not be initiated when clients are concurrently engaged in other therapies likely to compete for time and energy.

In general, OCD symptom severity does not factor into the decision of whether to use medication or ERP – we suggest ERP as the first-line treatment for any severity level. However, severe symptoms may require a more intense regimen of whatever treatment is offered – that is, a higher dose of medicine or more supervised ERP. If the client presents a danger to self or others, residential treatment might be recommended. Where possible, however, we recommend ERP be conducted on an outpatient basis to maximize generalizability of treatment gains to the client's own personal surroundings.

3.4.7 OCD Symptom Theme

Both ERP and medication can produce improvement across the various presentations of OCD (e.g., washing, checking). Although it is clinical lore that clients with obsessions and mental rituals (sometimes referred to as "pure obsessions") do not fare well in ERP, as we show in Chapter 4, ERP can indeed be adapted to successfully treat this presentation of OCD.

3.4.8 Interpersonal Factors

Consider involving a partner or family member in treatment

Accommodation of OCD symptoms by a partner, relative, or close friend is related to more severe obsessions and compulsions, as well as to poorer long-term treatment outcome. Similarly, interpersonal communication patterns characterized by criticism, hostility, and emotional overinvolvement are associated with premature treatment discontinuation and symptom relapse. On the other hand, communication patterns characterized by empathy, hopefulness, and assertiveness are associated with successful outcomes with ERP. Where accommodation and/or hostility are present, it is worth considering involving the partner or a family member in treatment to work on modifying these maladaptive communication patterns that maintain OCD symptoms. Before enlisting such a person, however, be sure they can interact in a supportive yet firm (i.e., assertive) way with the client. The ability to be firm yet relaxed and empathic is predictive of better results. Overinvolvement, hostility, and inconsistent behavior can lead to treatment attrition.

3.4.9 Insight

Clients with poorer insight into the senselessness of their OCD symptoms show an attenuated response to ERP due to (a) reluctance to engage in ERP and (b) difficulty consolidating what is to be learned from treatment. While ERP is worth attempting, increased use of cognitive therapy techniques might be necessary to help clients engage in (and benefit from) exposure tasks. Another augmentative approach is to use medication; some psychiatrists use antipsychotic medication to treat clients with very poor insight.

3.4.10 Comorbidity

Clients with comorbid depression or GAD show reduced response to ERP. Seriously depressed clients may become demoralized and have trouble complying with treatment instructions. Their strong negative affect may also exacerbate OCD symptoms. In GAD, pervasive worry detracts from clients' mental resources available for learning skills in ERP. The front-line treatment for both GAD and depression includes cognitive therapy, with the addition of behavioral activation for depressed clients; thus, a transdiagnostic approach could be adopted into treatment by adding these interventions into the treatment plan.

For clients with comorbid OCD and posttraumatic stress disorder (PTSD), there may be times in which these two conditions have become intertwined (e.g., clients who were sexually assaulted and now have obsessions about cleanliness and feeling dirty – what is sometimes referred to as *mental contamination*). In some cases, clients may benefit from concurrent work targeting both OCD and PTSD-related fears (e.g., a goal of an exposure exercise might be to touch a public restroom toilet, and then tolerate obsessions about getting sick, disgust about feeling "dirty," and memories of the trauma). In others, clients might pursue PTSD-focused treatment first before beginning ERP.

Other conditions likely to interfere with ERP are those that involve alterations in perception, cognition, and judgment, such as psychotic and manic symptoms. Clients actively abusing psychoactive substances are also poor ERP candidates. These problems impede the ability to profit from ERP exercises and can also reduce adherence. Similarly, clients with anorexia who are too far below the expected body weight for their age and height may not have the cognitive resources to be able to consolidate key information from doing ERP. Bringing these comorbid conditions under control is necessary before beginning ERP.

Both ERP and medication may be adversely affected by severe *personality disorder* (PD) psychopathology. Anxious (e.g., OCPD) and dramatic (e.g., histrionic) traits may interfere with rapport development; yet success is possible if a therapeutic relationship can be established. Clients with personality traits in the odd cluster (e.g., schizotypy) present a challenge to ERP due to their reduced ability to consolidate corrective information from exposure or cognitive interventions.

3.4.11 Treatment History

Clients who have received an adequate dosage of one or more SRIs for a reasonable length of time (at least 12 weeks) without a response are generally unlikely to respond to other SRIs or to combinations of SRIs. Thus, for medicated clients who have not had psychological treatment, ERP is the logical recommendation. If clients report that they have undergone CBT, assess the adequacy of the previous trial before making additional recommendations. If therapy sessions were infrequent, or if therapist-guided exposure was not incorporated, a course of consistent therapist-supervised ERP should be considered. On the other hand, a history of adherence problems may suggest the need for residential treatment or a supportive approach.

3.5 Presenting the Recommendation for ERP

How to recommend ERP to the client

Once you have determined that a client is a candidate for ERP, present a summary of the assessment results and a rationale for starting treatment. At the client's discretion, close friends or family members (e.g., spouse, partner, or parent) who can be counted on to provide support can be included in this discussion. Convey the following points during this consultation:

- Review the data collected during the interview which suggest the presence (and severity level) of OCD.
- Define OCD and review the signs and symptoms as discussed in Section 1.2. Use the client's own symptoms as examples. Emphasize that OCD is a chronic problem that is unlikely to get better without effective treatment.

- Explain that the exact causes of OCD are unknown and that, most likely, numerous factors (biological and environmental) are involved.
- Explain that effective treatment does not require that we know the *causes*, but that we understand what *maintains* OCD symptoms (i.e., understanding the link between obsessions, compulsions, and how they work). Fortunately, after much research, we understand these symptoms and how they maintain each other very well.
- Describe ERP as a form of treatment in which the client learns skills to (a) more effectively respond to and manage fear-provoking situations and unwanted obsessional thoughts, (b) reduce avoidance behavior and compulsive rituals, and (c) improve quality of life.
- Using the information in Section 3.3 as a guide, describe the ERP procedures. Provide examples of the kinds of exposure exercises and response prevention strategies that might be used in treatment.
- Explain that during treatment the client can expect to experience anxiety and distress, but that with guided practice, they will learn how to relate to and manage this anxiety in healthier ways so that they can live their life without being "bullied" by OCD. Suggestions for how to convey this might include: "You will develop a healthier relationship with anxiety and obsessional thoughts so they have less of a hold on you and aren't so 'loud' in your mind" and "The object of treatment is not so much to make anxiety go away forever, which is impossible, but rather to be 'better' at making room for anxiety when it does occur."
- Assure the client that you realize treatment will be hard work, but that you believe in their ability to be successful and rise to the challenge. Review the advantages and disadvantages to this approach.
- Use the analogy of the therapist as a *coach*: you will work collaboratively with the client to help them learn and practice a set of skills. You will never *force* them to do an exercise they do not want to do, but instead will challenge them to push themselves in ERP.
- Ensure the client understands that how much they benefit from ERP is related to how much effort they put into doing the treatment.
- Recommend a trial of 16 sessions of ERP and answer any questions from the client (and family members).

Treatment

4.1 Methods of Treatment

The "nuts and bolts" of conducting ERP

This chapter presents the fundamentals of how to plan and implement ERP for OCD. Box 3 shows a suggested agenda for what is to be accomplished in each treatment session, although flexibility is encouraged to adapt to the unique needs and progress of each client. Treatment might be delivered in once-weekly, twice-weekly, or even daily sessions depending on symptom severity and access issues (e.g., clients traveling from out of town might receive five daily sessions for 3 consecutive weeks).

Box 3 Suggested Session Structure in ERP for OCD
Session 1
• Begin functional assessment of OCD symptoms • Introduce self-monitoring • Begin psychoeducation
Session 2
• Continue functional assessment • Psychoeducation • Informal cognitive therapy • Begin planning for exposure and generating the exposure list
Session 3
• Psychoeducation • Informal cognitive therapy • Finalize and agree on the exposure treatment plan
Sessions 4–14
• Exposure • Response prevention • Informal cognitive therapy
Sessions 15 & 16
• Final exposures • Relapse prevention • Wrapping up exposure and response prevention • Assess outcome

Research and clinical experience also suggests that in many instances, delivering treatment virtually or remotely (or using a hybrid approach) is as effective as in-person appointments (see Section 4.4.4).

4.1.1 Functional Assessment

Functional assessment – the collecting of detailed, client-specific information

Functional assessment is the collection of highly detailed client-specific information about obsessional triggers and the cognitive and behavioral responses to these stimuli, including a complete description of all compulsive rituals and avoidance strategies (behavioral and mental). The cognitive-behavioral model dictates what information is collected and how it is organized to form an individualized conceptualization of the problem and treatment plan. The *Functional Assessment of OCD Symptoms* form (see Appendix 1) is used to document this information. Depending on the complexity of the client's symptoms, this assessment might last from 1 to 3 hrs. Begin by providing a rationale for the detailed functional assessment that incorporates the following points:

- ERP involves learning skills to reduce OCD symptoms.
- To tailor the program to address the client's specific obsessions and rituals, it is important to have a thorough understanding of these symptoms.
- Treatment will therefore begin by generating a list of all the situations, thoughts, and other stimuli that evoke anxiety and urges to do rituals.

Assessing Obsessional Stimuli

Generate a comprehensive list of external triggers and internal stimuli (thoughts, body sensations) that evoke obsessional fear. These stimuli might later be used in exposure exercises.

External Triggers

Identify all objects, situations, places, etc. that evoke obsessional fear and urges to ritualize. Examples include bathrooms, knives, sending emails or text messages, churches, the number 13, leaving the house, driving in certain places, reading about serial killers, and so on. Examples of questions to elicit this information include:

- What kinds of situations make you feel anxious, guilty, disgusted, etc.?
- What situations make you feel uncertain about something that could go wrong?
- What prompts you to want to do rituals?
- What do you avoid because it triggers obsessions, anxiety, disgust, or rituals?

Obsessional Thoughts and Other Internal Triggers

In OCD, anxiety is also evoked by recurring intrusive ideas, images, doubts, and bodily sensations that the client finds upsetting, immoral, repulsive, or otherwise unacceptable. Examples include thoughts of germs and illness, ideas to vandalize a sacred place, unwanted images, ideas about loved ones being injured, doubts about making mistakes, uncertainty about things that are difficult to know for sure (e.g., "Am I going to heaven or hell when I die?"), and doubts about whether one has mistakenly caused physical or emotional harm to innocent people or loved ones. Feared body sensations might include an increased heart rate that could be caused by either sexual or anxious arousal. Examples of questions to elicit this information include:

- What intrusive thoughts, images, and doubts do you have that trigger fear, anxiety, or uncertainty?
- What thoughts do you try to avoid, resist, or dismiss?
- What body sensations do you experience that provoke fear and uncertainty?

Identify fears of disastrous consequences that are immediate, long-term, and "unknowable"

Assessing Cognitive Features

Obtain information about the following cognitive parameters of the client's fear.

Fairly Immediate Feared Consequences

Clients may articulate fears that something terrible will happen fairly immediately if they approach their obsessional stimuli or if they fail to perform certain rituals. For example, they would become ill, be responsible for harm befalling a loved one, snap and commit a violent act, experience bad luck from confronting the number 13, or make serious or costly mistakes (e.g., offend someone in a text). Examples of questions to elicit such feared consequences include:

- What do you fear would happen if you were to approach ______ (obsessional trigger)?
- What do you think might happen if you didn't do your ______ rituals?

Importantly, the idea is not to challenge these fears at this point. It is merely to understand them from the client's point of view.

Long-Term or "Unknowable" Feared Outcomes

Many people with OCD have feared consequences that might not materialize for a long time (e.g., many years). Examples include developing cancer someday, gradually evolving into a child molester, and being arrested by the police at some point for causing an automobile accident. Sometimes, the feared consequences are simply impossible to verify, such as "What if I go to hell when I die?" "What if I'm not disgusted enough when thinking about child abuse?" and "What if I'm in a dream and nothing really exists?" These types of feared consequences are driven by an intolerance of uncertainty, and questions to elicit them include:

- What is the worst part about having these thoughts?
- What is the worst thing you imagine might happen as a result of this situation in the future?
- What terrible things that could happen to you later on do your rituals help to prevent?
- If you don't do your rituals correctly, what do you worry about most in the future?

Misinterpretations of Obsessional Thoughts

Identify mistaken beliefs about the presence and meaning of intrusive obsessional thoughts and images. For example, "Thinking about stabbing my wife could lead me to actually stab her," "God will punish me for thinking immoral thoughts," "I'm a pervert if I have unwanted thoughts about sex," and "I couldn't function at work if I'm having this thought." Examples of questions to elicit this information include:

Identify how the client misinterprets obsessional thoughts

- What do you think it means that you have this thought?
- What are you afraid might happen if you just let yourself have this thought?
- Why do you try to avoid or dismiss these thoughts?

Fears of Experiencing Long-Term Anxiety, Uncertainty, and Incompleteness

Some clients fear that anxiety (and arousal-related bodily sensations) will persist indefinitely, spiral out of control, or cause other catastrophic consequences (e.g., physical harm) if allowed to continue without rituals or avoidance. This is often based on the belief that anxiety is intolerable or even harmful. In the same vein, clients sometimes describe the fear that uncertainty and doubt associated with an obsession (e.g., fears of "snapping" and committing murder) will continue indefinitely and become unbearable. Finally, clients with ordering and arranging compulsions may describe a sense of imperfection or incompleteness (also known as "not-just-right experiences") that they fear will persist or become intolerable if allowed to continue without performing rituals. Questions to help elicit these types of fears include:

Some clients instead worry that anxiety and uncertainty will persist indefinitely

- Do you worry that you will become anxious and that the anxiety will never go away?
- What might happen to you if you remained uncertain about this obsession?
- Do you worry that feelings of imperfection or incompleteness will stay with you forever?

Some clients have difficulty articulating these types of fears and might require prompting to be able to describe such concerns (e.g., "Some people with OCD have the fear that if they don't ritualize, their anxiety will go on endlessly and become unbearable. Do you worry about this?").

Assessing Distress-Reduction Behaviors

It is important to know about all of the client's responses to obsessional thoughts and fears (i.e., avoidance strategies, neutralizing, safety-seeking rituals, etc.), that serve to reduce or control unacceptable thoughts and distress. Such behaviors maintain OCD, interfere with functioning, and need to be targeted in response prevention. In addition, the mere *availability* of safety cues and the *possibility* of performing distress-reducing behaviors should be taken into account; such as a client reminding herself that she could always use the hand sanitizer stored in her car if her anxiety became "too intense."

Determine the client's maladaptive response to obsessional fear

Passive Avoidance

Most clients avoid situations and objects associated with obsessions in order to prevent feared disasters. Examples include avoidance of certain people (e.g., cancer patients), objects (e.g., knives), places (e.g., public washrooms), situations (e.g., using social media, bathing one's infant), and certain words (e.g., "devil" or "suicide"). Pay particular attention to subtle avoidance habits such as staying away from the most used surface (for fear of germs) or refraining from listening to music while driving (for fear of being distracted and causing harm). Ascertain the cognitive basis for avoidance (e.g., "If I touch the most used surface of the table, I will be more likely to get sick" or "If I go on social media, I might post something inappropriate or offensive by mistake"). Examples of questions to elicit this information include:

- What situations do you avoid because of obsessional fear?
- Is there anything that you procrastinate or put off because it will generate anxiety or lead to time-consuming rituals?
- Can you ever confront this situation? Under what circumstances?
- How does avoiding ______ make you feel more comfortable?

Overt Compulsive Rituals

List all ritualistic behaviors including cleaning, checking, repeating actions, arranging objects, and asking for reassurance. Attend to inconspicuous behaviors such as subtle wiping, the use of special soaps, and excessive inspection (e.g., for signs of contamination). Finally, assess the relationship between rituals and feared consequences. For example, using a certain brand soap *to target a certain type of germ* and repeating a behavior such as turning on a light switch *until a certain thought has been dismissed*. Examples of questions to elicit this information include:

- What do you do when you can't avoid ______ (insert situation)?
- Tell me about the strategies or rituals you use to reduce fear of ______ (insert obsessional fear).
- How does doing this ritual reduce your discomfort?
- What might happen if you didn't engage in this ritual?

Mental Rituals and Covert Distress-Reduction Strategies

Inquire about mental rituals and other covert neutralizing strategies

Inquire about the use of mental rituals to control or neutralize obsessional thoughts. Examples include thinking special "safe" thoughts, phrases, and images to replace "dangerous" ones; repeating prayers in a set (or "perfect") way; mentally reviewing (over and over) one's actions to allay obsessional doubts; self-reassurance that feared outcomes won't occur; and habitual thought suppression and mental distraction. Ascertain the client's rationale for performing mental rituals (e.g., repeating the phrase "God is good" to avoid punishment for having sacrilegious thoughts; distracting oneself from violent thoughts to prevent acting violently). Clients may not spontaneously report these strategies without prompting (as they may not recognize them as distinct from obsessional thoughts). Thus, it may be beneficial to ask about them directly. Examples of questions to elicit this information include:

- What kinds of mental strategies do you use to control or dismiss unwanted thoughts?
- How do you deal with your upsetting thoughts in your mind?
- What might happen if you didn't use these strategies?
- Many people with OCD will try to ______ (insert mental ritual) when they have an unwanted thought. Is that something you do?

Symptom Accommodation

For clients in close relationships, and those living with friends or family members, it is important to assess how others might be accommodating OCD symptoms. Such accommodation will need to be addressed during treatment. It might be helpful to include significant others (e.g., partner or spouse, parent, adult child) in the assessment session to collect this information. Some suggested questions for clients and their loved ones to help identify problematic relationship patterns concerning OCD symptoms include the following:

- Tell me about the ways OCD affects your relationship with ______.
- Between you and ______, what patterns have developed because of OCD symptoms?
- How have you tried to cope with ______'s OCD symptoms?
- How do you, as a couple (or as a family) manage situations when ______ is experiencing obsessional fear or doing rituals? Does it ever lead to anger or arguments? What happens in these situations?
- When ______ is having problems with OCD, how do other people respond? Do they help reduce ______'s anxiety, avoid situations, or assist with compulsive rituals?
- Tell me about how the two of you (or your family) communicate about the OCD problem.

Assessing the Effects of OCD Symptoms on Quality of Life

OCD symptoms – especially compulsive rituals and excessive avoidance – typically lead to disruption in one or more areas of functioning. Assess how this plays out for the client, noting even seemingly minor areas of interference. The following questions are helpful to assess functional interference in important life domains:

- How does OCD get in the way of being successful at work or school?
- What kinds of problems do you have in your relationships because of OCD?
- How does OCD keep you from enjoying the things in life that you would like to enjoy?
- In what ways does OCD keep you from being as physically and emotionally healthy as you would like to be?

Clinical Pearl
The Play-by-Play Description of a Typical Episode

To gain additional insight into the client's experience, you can ask for a "play-by-play" description of a few specific instances of obsessional fear, avoidance, and rituals. This technique could also be used to focus the assessment on a particular symptom you are having difficulty understanding. It involves asking questions such as, "Tell me about the situation that triggered the obsessional fear; what was the first sign of trouble?" Then, ask the client to walk you through the episode and report what they were thinking and feeling. How distressed or anxious did the client become, and what did they do to reduce this anxiety (i.e., ask for a detailed description of the rituals, avoidance, etc.)? How did the situation resolve itself, and how did they feel afterwards? You can also point out the relationships between obsessions and increased distress, and how rituals or avoidance reduce anxiety. Illustrating to the client how these symptoms are related (as opposed to being bizarre or "out of control") can instill hope in the therapy program, as well as a sense of trust in your expertise.

4.1.2 Self-Monitoring

Self-monitoring is an important (and often overlooked) component of ERP

To aid the functional assessment, ask the client to use the *Self-Monitoring of OCD Rituals* form (see Appendix 2) to keep a real-time log of situations and thoughts that lead to rituals between sessions. During the first session, explain the form's importance and give instructions for completing it. Some clients do not carefully and accurately self-monitor because they do not appreciate the task's relevance to treatment (many see it as "busy work"). To increase adherence, convey the following:

- Self-monitoring helps both the therapist and the client gain an accurate picture of the time spent engaged in, and situations that lead to, rituals.
- It helps the client identify obsessions and rituals that they might not be aware of.
- Some clients use the fact that they have to record their rituals as motivation to resist them (i.e., so they don't have to write anything down).
- Accurate reporting of rituals between now and the end of treatment will help track how much progress is made in therapy.

With the client's input, choose which rituals will be monitored (i.e., the most prominent ones). Then, give the following instructions:

- Rather than guess, use a watch or timer to determine the exact amount of time spent ritualizing.
- To avoid forgetting important details, record each ritual *immediately*, rather than waiting until the end of the day (or worse, right before the next session).
- Write a *brief* summary of the situation or thought that evoked the ritual.
- Log *subjective units of distress* (SUDS; 0–100) that you experienced before giving into the ritual. For more details on this scale see Section 4.1.6.

- Record any details about how the rituals ended up interfering with your quality of life (e.g., a 15-minute checking ritual might result in your missing your bus to work and arriving late to a meeting).

In the session, practice self-monitoring one or two recent rituals to make sure the client understands how to use the form. To further increase adherence, explain that the first item on the agenda for the next session will be to review this form (and make sure to stick to this promise!).

4.1.3 Psychoeducation

Psychoeducation helps socialize the client to the cognitive-behavioral approach to OCD

The educational component of ERP helps lay the foundation for moving forward in treatment. You will help the client understand their OCD symptoms through a cognitive-behavioral lens to maximize treatment effectiveness. You will also explain that the purpose of ERP is not primarily to *reduce* distress, but to help the client learn to approach and manage anxiety, uncertainty, guilt, disgust, etc. without struggling so intensely against it – an approach that supports long-term progress. The specific concepts to be conveyed are (a) the symptoms and patterns involved in OCD are well-understood; (b) unwanted intrusive thoughts, doubts, disgust, and anxiety are universal experiences, and as such, they are safe and manageable; (c) misinterpretations of intrusive thoughts lead to obsessional fear and preoccupation; (d) avoidance and compulsive rituals are attempts to control distress, but they do not work and instead make obsessions worse; and (e) treatment is based on this way of thinking about OCD. Presenting a coherent rationale is especially important since clients who do not see how ERP ultimately produces benefit cannot be expected to fully engage in these challenging techniques.

Understanding the Symptoms of OCD

Explain the functional relationship between obsessions and rituals

Use the points below to begin with an explanation of OCD as involving three components. Include examples from the functional assessment to illustrate these points:

- A good way to think about OCD is that it has three parts.
- The first part is the *unwanted inner experiences*, such as unwelcome thoughts (obsessions) about ______, feelings of anxiety, fear, guilt, or disgust about ______, uncertainty and doubt about ______, a sense of incompleteness or imperfection, or other unpleasant body sensations (e.g., racing heart). These experiences tend to show up without your choosing or inviting them.
- The second part of OCD is the *strategies you use to try to control or get rid of these unwanted inner experiences*, such as by avoiding ______ and doing compulsive rituals like ______. These behaviors are mostly within your control, although it doesn't always seem that way.
- Next, begin a discussion about *how the strategies work* (or *don't* work!) to alleviate unwanted inner experiences. You might ask the client to describe their strategies and their short- and long-term effects. The point of this discussion is to help the client realize that although the strategies may

sometimes *temporarily* work, they are not good long-term solutions since the obsessions and anxiety always find a way to come back. Additionally, the more the client uses these strategies, the more compulsive behaviors they end up needing to perform to manage their distress. So, the client ends up spending a great deal of time and energy on these counterproductive behaviors.

- The third part of OCD is the *disruption in your life*, such as how problems with OCD interfere with daily routines, work, leisure, social functioning, relationships, etc.
- It is important to keep in mind that it is the strategies in Part 2 (not so much the inner experiences in Part 1) that most directly cause the disruption in daily functioning. For example, it's the *checking rituals* (not the obsessional thoughts about mistakes) that lead to lateness or missing deadlines; and the *avoidance of public places* (not anxiety about germs) that leads to missing out on going to the movies.
- Given that avoidance and compulsions are easier to control than obsessions, and that the negative effects on quality of life are generally the product of (futile) attempts to avoid, resist, and control obsessional thoughts and other unpleasant inner experiences (rather than these experiences themselves), treatment for OCD will foster new ways to interact with obsessions, uncertainty, disgust, and anxiety, in order to lessen the need to engage in avoidance and rituals. This, in turn, will improve overall quality of life.

The next sections provide ideas and suggestions for how to present authoritative information about OCD and its treatment to help the client become more acquainted with the cognitive-behavioral approach.

Normalizing Obsessional Thoughts and Other Unwanted Inner Experiences

Everyone has obsessional thoughts

Explain that unwanted, senseless, or bizarre intrusive (obsessional) thoughts, ideas, or images are a key part of OCD. Sometimes these thoughts are sparked by external stimuli (e.g., knives, movie scenes), whereas at other times they may be unprovoked. Similarly, the experiences of anxiety (on an emotional and a physiological level) and uncertainty are ever-present in OCD. Research shows that unwanted thoughts (no matter how repugnant or upsetting) are common experiences for over 90% of the population, and that these thoughts are usually not under our control (Rachman & Hodgson, 1980). People with OCD frequently misinterpret these kinds of thoughts as very significant and meaningful, whereas people without OCD simply consider them (correctly) as "mental noise." As the therapist, it can be helpful to share examples of your own intrusive thoughts to demonstrate that these experiences are universal, and to model acceptance of them as part of human existence. Clients may be surprised (and relieved) to find out that just about everyone has unwanted intrusive thoughts – including their therapist.

If the client wants to know *why* people have strange or unwanted thoughts in the first place, explain that the brain is capable of enormous creativity.

People can imagine all kinds of scenarios – pleasant and unpleasant. For example, many people daydream of winning the lottery or scoring the winning touchdown in the Superbowl. Just as our *thought generator* produces positive thoughts that are unlikely to come true, it can also produce unpleasant thoughts that are equally improbable.

Explain that anxiety is also a fundamental part of being human. In fact, all animals experience anxiety and fear as part of their *fight-or-flight response* when they perceive threat. The purpose of anxiety is to protect animals (including humans) from danger. In other words, we need anxiety – it is our friend. We often feel most anxious about the things that matter to us (i.e., the things that we value) – thus, anxiety reveals to us what is most important to us in life. That said, it can produce unpleasant physiological (e.g., racing heart, shortness of breath), emotional (e.g., racing thoughts, apprehension), and behavioral (e.g., restlessness, urge to escape) experiences. It is important to remember that despite their unpleasantness, these experiences serve a protective function (e.g., the heart races to pump blood to the body's muscles) to keep us safe from danger.

Dysfunctional beliefs and interpretations give rise to emotional distress

In OCD, however, the perceived threats that trigger the anxiety response are not actually dangerous – they generally pose no more than ordinary everyday risk (e.g., flushing the toilet, using the oven, thinking of something upsetting). Thus, obsessional anxiety can be viewed as a false alarm. It is important for clients to think of anxiety and fear as fundamentally helpful (i.e., the fight-or-flight response) and not inherently dangerous. For additional details on how to discuss this with clients, the reader is referred to the guide to the treatment of panic disorder by Craske and Barlow (2006).

Discuss with the client that fact that uncertainty is also a constant and unavoidable part of life, as it's nearly impossible to be completely certain about almost anything. People with OCD, however, often struggle to tolerate even ordinary levels of doubt and uncertainty – especially related to their obsessions. While most people accept everyday risks (e.g., using the oven without repeated checking), those with OCD may engage in excessive checking, reassurance-seeking, or other rituals in an effort to achieve an unrealistic level of certainty or safety. Overcoming OCD involves learning to accept and manage the normal, everyday uncertainty that is part of life.

Thus, underscore that the problem in OCD is not the occurrence of obsessional thoughts, anxiety, and uncertainty per se (remember that these are normal and universal experiences), but rather how the person *relates to* these experiences and perceives them as threatening. The aim of treatment is therefore not to eliminate obsessional thoughts, anxiety, and uncertainty, but rather to change one's relationship to these experiences. Once the client changes their stance toward these experiences and is more open and accepting of them, it will not matter as much when or how frequently they occur, and there will be less need for rituals. Give the client the *Everyone Has Intrusive Thoughts* handout (see Appendix 3) to be read after the session is over. The handout reviews this didactic information and includes a list of intrusive thoughts reported by people without OCD.

Clients may point out that although everyone has intrusive thoughts, their own intrusions are more frequent, more distressing, and more intense compared with those of people without OCD. This may be true, and it is therefore important for them to understand the role of thinking patterns (which they can learn to change) in causing normal intrusive thoughts to escalate into highly distressing and recurrent obsessions, as is discussed in the next section.

Role of Dysfunctional Thoughts and Beliefs in OCD

Helping the client understand the relationship between thoughts and emotions

At the heart of ERP is the idea that our emotions and behaviors are largely determined by our *thoughts and beliefs* about situations, not by the situations themselves. Accordingly, it is helpful for clients to understand the process by which their own mistaken thoughts and beliefs lead to emotional responses such as anxiety, which in turn, exacerbates obsessional thinking.

For example, when someone with obsessions about germs drops an object on the floor and then picks it up, the following dysfunctional (i.e., exaggerated, mistaken, or rigid) thoughts and beliefs might be activated: "Floors have lots of dangerous germs," "I am highly susceptible to illness", "I could get very sick", and "I've got be completely certain that I won't get sick." These cognitions evoke distress and the urge to ritualize (i.e., washing and cleaning).

Clinical Vignette 1 illustrates the use of a Socratic dialog in which the therapist helps the client understand how their thinking dictates their emotional and behavioral responses.

Clinical Vignette 1

Illustration of the Cognitive Model With Non-OCD-Relevant Situation

Therapist: Suppose you and a friend plan to meet for dinner at 7:00 p.m., and it is now 7:30 p.m. and your friend hasn't shown up or even called to say that she'll be late. If you conclude that your friend decided that you are no fun to be with, how will you feel?

Client: Sad or depressed.

Therapist: Right. How about if you believed your friend was being late on purpose and was being inconsiderate of your time?

Client: Then I'd feel angry.

Therapist: Sure. How about if you thought that your friend had been in a terrible accident?

Client: I'd be worried.

Therapist: Exactly. Do you see the importance of your thinking?

Client: Yes. Depending on how I interpret the same situation, I could feel different emotions.

Therapist: That's right. The way you think about situations influences your emotional responses. So, *you*, not situations, have control over your emotions. This is called the cognitive model of emotions.

After illustrating this model using a situation that is not emotionally charged for the client, the next step is to apply it to an OCD-relevant situation (Clinical Vignette 2). The client in the example had an excessive fear that she would catch the herpes virus from a particular coworker who once had a cold sore on her lip.

Clinical Vignette 2
Illustration of the Cognitive Model With OCD-Relevant Situation

Therapist: Now, let's see how the cognitive model might apply to OCD situations. You said that you become anxious and feel like washing your hands and changing your clothes whenever you are near this coworker. What kinds of thoughts go through your mind that might lead you to feel so anxious that you have to do these rituals?

Client: I think that cold sores are easy to get from other people, so I assume I would probably get a cold sore if I came anywhere near her. On the other hand, if I wash and change, I won't get any cold sores.

Therapist: Do you see how your assumptions about the probability of you getting a cold sore lead to anxiety and the urge to do compulsive behaviors to prevent cold sores?

Client: Yes, I see that.

Therapist: You said that other people don't wash themselves or change after interacting with this coworker. What must they be assuming about cold sores to keep them from feeling anxious or from having to do these rituals?

Client: They probably don't think about it; or they just assume they won't get a cold sore unless there's intimate contact.

Therapist: Yes, that would make sense. Can you see that if you learned to think the same way, your coworker wouldn't seem so threatening anymore, and you wouldn't feel like you had to ritualize to stay safe?

Client: I understand, but I can't just change my mind. I mean, I'm better safe than sorry, right!?

Therapist: That's what therapy is going to help you with. We're going to work together to help you learn how to get through these kinds of situations in ways that will be more effective for you. In other words, we'll start making behavioral changes that will in time result in changes in how you think about situations such as interacting with your coworker. For now, though, it is important that you see how the cognitive model works. Your thinking patterns are what lead to your obsessions and anxiety.

In OCD the mistaken beliefs and assumptions are often about intrusive (obsessional) thoughts, rather than about situations. Applying the cognitive model with thoughts as triggers can be tricky since these stimuli, and the maladaptive thoughts and beliefs, are all mental events. Help the client to distinguish between (a) intrusive obsessional thoughts and (b) thoughts and beliefs *about* these intrusions, as in Clinical Vignette 3. The client in this vignette was devoutly religious, yet experienced unwanted sacrilegious thoughts such as "God is the devil's bitch" and "Jesus sucks." He interpreted these thoughts as meaning that despite a seemingly strong devotion to God, he was actually a fraud (and devil worshipper). This provoked obsessional doubts about his salvation and constant prayer and reassurance-seeking rituals.

Clinical Vignette 3

Distinguishing Between Intrusive Obsessional Thoughts and Dysfunctional Beliefs

Therapist: You said that when these thoughts come to mind, you become uncertain about your faith and salvation, tell yourself that you are a fraud, try to stop yourself from thinking these thoughts, pray for forgiveness, and seek reassurance that you are still a Christian. Can you see how you are interpreting your unwanted thoughts as very threatening?

Client: Yes, I see that.

Therapist: What emotions do those threatening interpretations lead to? What do they make you do?

Client: They make me feel anxious and guilty, so I avoid churches, and I am always praying to make sure I'm still saved.

Therapist: Right. So, the question is, Do these unwanted and senseless thoughts really mean you are not a Christian and that you're not saved? We might not have the answers to these questions, but is it possible to be a faithful Christian even without a 100% guarantee of salvation? Does anyone really have a 100% guarantee of certainty that they're saved? Isn't that what having faith is all about?

Client: Well, if, like you said, most people have unwanted thoughts about things that distress them, and if it's impossible to have a guarantee about things like faith and salvation, I guess you would say these thoughts and doubts are not really the problem. But that seems strange. I've worried about those thoughts and feelings for so long.

Therapist: That's because you have believed for a long time that those thoughts are very important and that you need to have a guarantee of your salvation. But actually, these thoughts and doubts are not even consistent with how you really feel about your religion. Everyone now and then has ideas that conflict with their personal beliefs and morals. Everyone experiences doubts at some point. In therapy, you will learn healthier ways to respond to these kinds of thoughts and doubts, so that you are better able to practice your faith the way you want to.

Role of Avoidance, Rituals, and Other Distress-Reduction Strategies in Maintaining OCD

Explain how safety-seeking beaviors maintain obsessional fear

Help clients understand how their avoidance, rituals, and other attempts to reduce or control unpleasant inner experiences (e.g., thought suppression) contribute to the vicious cycle of OCD. This will provide a rationale for response prevention. Discuss the following points:

- Review how obsessions increase anxiety, and compulsive rituals temporarily decrease anxiety.
- Aside from compulsive rituals, there are other strategies that people often use that have the same effects as rituals. These include avoidance, subtle (mini) rituals, seeking reassurance, and thought suppression attempts.
- Avoidance and rituals might seem strange, bizarre, or "uncontrollable." Help the client view them as deliberate distress-reduction strategies.

Give an example of how rituals are used to neutralize obsessional anxiety or provide reassurance. Make sure the functional relationship between obsessions and compulsions is understood.

- Rituals would be adaptive responses if there were actual danger present. But obsessional fear is based on mistaken beliefs and interpretations about situations and inner experiences (e.g., intrusive thoughts) that objectively pose little risk. So, these responses are unnecessary and counterproductive.
- Avoidance prevents clients from learning that their feared situations are not especially dangerous, and that the anxiety and uncertainty associated with situations and obsessional thoughts is manageable.
- When obsessional stimuli cannot be avoided, the next best solution seems like *escaping* from the feared situation and relieving the anxiety, uncertainty, guilt, and/or disgust as quickly as possible in any way that seems to work (provide examples of how the client's rituals are used to escape from obsessional fear). But this is a trap because the fact that these escape strategies sometimes temporarily reduce distress makes them develop into compulsive rituals that are difficult to stop.
- In summary, strategies used to avoid, control, or escape from obsessional thoughts, anxiety, disgust and uncertainty often seem helpful in the moment, but backfire in the long run since the obsessions and anxiety always return. Not only that, these strategies also take up time, interfere with relationships, and interfere with important areas of the client's life.
- Treatment will weaken these patterns by creating opportunities for the client to learn that they can manage the unpleasant inner experiences and anxiety-provoking situations without avoiding, ritualizing, or using other control strategies.

Clinical Pearl

Integrating Psychoeducation Into the Functional Assessment

A useful way to think about the initial sessions of ERP is as an exchange of information between client and therapist. On the one hand, the client is an "expert" regarding their particular OCD symptoms and will need to help the therapist understand the nuances of these symptoms so that an individual treatment plan can be developed. On the other hand, the therapist is an expert in conceptualizing OCD symptoms and needs to teach the client to understand their symptoms in a way that best fosters benefit from the treatment procedures.

We recommend explaining this relationship at the very beginning of the functional assessment phase. We then weave the psychoeducational component into this assessment by capitalizing on any opportunities to help the client understand the functional aspects of their symptoms. For example, when assessing obsessional thoughts, if a client describes intrusive thoughts as "strange" or "abnormal," or insinuates that they are the only person with such thoughts, we supply education about the normalcy of unwanted thoughts. This helps socialize the client to the cognitive-behavioral model of OCD, which is critical for a positive treatment response.

Presenting the Rationale for ERP and Explaining the Process

Once the client has a grasp of the cognitive-behavioral model, present a rationale for ERP by discussing the following points:

- The treatment techniques, *exposure and response prevention*, are designed to teach the client that (a) obsessional thoughts, anxiety, guilt, disgust, and uncertainty – although unpleasant – are safe and manageable; and (b) the use of rituals and other distress-reduction strategies, which interfere with quality of life, are unnecessary. You *could* merely discuss these issues with the client, but ERP provides real life experiential evidence, which is more convincing than just talking (as we like to put it, "experience is the best teacher").
- Exposure involves engaging with situations and thoughts that evoke obsessional anxiety and doubt. Response prevention involves refraining from doing anything to avoid, reduce, or control these internal experiences.
- Use information from the functional assessment to give examples of specific exposure and response preventions exercises that might be used to help the client learn that obsessional thoughts, uncertainty, disgust and the situations that evoke these experiences are safe and manageable.

How to explain the concepts of habituation and anxiety acceptance

- One basic idea of exposure therapy is that repeatedly approaching and engaging with situations and thoughts that evoke obsessional anxiety and uncertainty helps the client learn that the anxiety and uncertainty will not persist indefinitely or spiral to out of control levels. In fact, the distress will subside naturally over time even without any rituals – a process called *habituation.*
- Another important idea behind exposure is that it teaches clients that anxiety and uncertainty are safe and manageable regardless of how long they take to subside. In other words, it helps clients become better at experiencing anxiety without trying to control or avoid it – a process called *anxiety acceptance*. Thus, *habituation is not required for exposure to be successful.*
- Since the client has usually avoided or escaped from the obsessional distress by doing rituals, they have not had the opportunity to consistently practice *leaning in* to these experiences and discovering that they are safe and manageable. ERP provides this opportunity to develop self-confidence and self-efficacy in one's ability to approach these experiences.

The client should understand that treatment is tailored to their specific OCD symptoms

Next, discuss what is likely to happen during exposure as follows:

- The client should expect to feel anxious, uncertain, disgusted, etc., especially when starting to approach the feared situation. But if the client stays in the situation without trying to control these feelings, one of two things will happen: The feelings will either begin to subside on their own, or they will remain present and the client will discover that they can manage the distress, even if it feels unpleasant.
- This learning only occurs if the exposure exercise is carefully designed, the client fully engages without performing rituals, and the practice is repeated consistently across various situations (e.g., office, home, in public).

- Two kinds of exposure are typically used in the treatment of OCD: *Situational* or *in vivo* exposure means engaging with the actual feared situations. *Imaginal exposure* means approaching fears and doubts in imagination and can be used either in conjunction with in vivo exposure (e.g., touching a public restroom toilet and then imaging a future illness one might contract) or for feared consequences that would not be safe or ethical to tackle in real life (e.g., burning down one's home).
- ERP is likely to be very helpful, but it requires consistent effort and the client needs to be properly coached in order to get meaningful results.

Next, discuss how you will work with the client to tailor the treatment program to their needs.

- The client and therapist will collaboratively create a to-do list of exposure stimuli that will include moderately anxiety-provoking situations up to those that are more difficult.
- The exposure stimuli do not need to be approached in any particular order. They might be addressed hierarchically (i.e., beginning with easier stimuli and working up to more distressing ones), or according to the client's priorities, or based on how much overcoming the fear would improve the client's quality of life.
- The therapist will provide support and coaching during each exposure task in the session, and the client will be asked to practice exposures on their own between sessions.
- Sometimes, exposure might *seem* risky or involve doing (or thinking about) things that most people would not ordinarily do (or think about) on purpose (e.g., a suggested exposure exercise might be to eat off the floor, which a client might point out is something that most people do not typically do). Yet the purpose of ERP is not just to practice doing what *most people* do. Exposure tasks are designed to foster new learning: that the feared situations are safe and/or that the inner experiences of obsessional thoughts, anxiety, disgust, and uncertainty are also safe and manageable. Accordingly, sometimes going above and beyond will help prepare clients for when challenges come up in their day-to-day life (e.g., they drop something important on the floor by accident).

The relationship between client and therapist in ERP is almost like that between a student and a teacher, or between an athlete and a coach. In the example below, the therapist explained his role as similar to that of a music teacher (Clinical Vignette 4).

The therapist is essentially the client's coach for overcoming OCD

Clinical Vignette 4

Describing the Client–Therapist Relationship

The best way to think of me is as your coach. Let's say you wanted to learn to play a musical instrument like the drums. You would go to a drum teacher who would give you instructions and then watch you play to look for things that you need to work on. The teacher would then help you improve your technique and suggest that you practice hard between lessons. Now, if you didn't practice the new techniques, or if you practiced them in a different way from how the teacher taught you, you would not develop the skills needed to be a good drummer. Also, the teacher would not force you to practice – you would decide whether or not to practice. If you didn't practice, the teacher might encourage you to practice more, but eventually they might stop the lessons if it was clear that you weren't practicing enough.

Treatment for OCD goes the same way. We'll work together to design exposure therapy exercises that will help you make progress in overcoming OCD. I'll guide you through how to approach them in a way that maximizes their effectiveness. The more consistently you practice them as we've planned, the more likely you are to see meaningful improvement. On the other hand, if the exercises aren't practiced regularly or are modified too much, progress may be slower than you'd like.

I have a great deal of confidence in this treatment and will work as hard as I can to help you – but you'll have to work even harder than me to get the real benefits you're looking for. I will challenge you and sometimes suggest things that feel difficult, but I will never force you. That said, I wouldn't be doing this with you if I didn't think that you're strong and can do the challenging work. I believe in you. I'll never ask you to do anything that you can't do. I'll also say up front that although they're unpleasant, your feared situations, obsessional thoughts, and anxiety are safe – which means they might not be 100% risk free, but any risk they do carry is acceptable – you can get through them. We are on the same team against OCD. If you do the hard work in therapy, you are likely to find that my coaching and support is very helpful.

4.1.4 Using Cognitive Therapy Techniques

Cognitive therapy techniques can be integrated informally into treatment

Cognitive therapy techniques for OCD teach clients to evaluate and modify maladaptive thinking patterns that give rise to obsessional fear and compulsive urges. This approach can help facilitate assessment, prevent premature discontinuation, and maximize adherence with ERP (Kozak & Coles, 2005), but we do not suggest using cognitive therapy techniques completely on their own (i.e., without exposure). Rather, we use these strategies informally throughout treatment in the context of ERP, often to reinforce what clients learn during exposure exercises. The primary style within cognitive therapy is the *Socratic dialog* in which the therapist promotes the client's learning by asking questions and making comments to facilitate independent, reflective, and critical thinking. Clinical Vignette 5 illustrates this type of dialogue, which is distinguished from didactic (i.e., lecture style) presentation of information (see Clinical Vignette 5). Ways of integrating cognitive therapy when OCD-related dysfunctional beliefs are present are discussed below.

Clinical Vignette 5
Example of Socratic Dialog

Therapist: So, you avoid eating at restaurants because you're worried about getting food poisoning?
Client: Yes. I can't help but think the food might be contaminated, and I'll get really sick.
Therapist: What do you think would happen if you did get food poisoning?
Client: I'd be very ill, probably end up in the hospital, and it would be a terrible experience.
Therapist: Have you ever gotten food poisoning from a restaurant before?
Client: No, but I've heard stories about people who have, and it scares me.
Therapist: How often do you find yourself thinking about this fear of food poisoning when you consider eating out?
Client: Almost every time. I can't enjoy the idea of dining out because I'm too focused on the potential risks.
Therapist: Do your friends or family have the same worries about eating at restaurants?
Client: No, they don't seem to worry about it at all. They eat out regularly and seem to enjoy it.
Therapist: Oh... So, your friends and family must get food poisoning a lot, right?
Client: [thinks] ... No, they don't.
Therapist: Interesting. What do you think it means if your friends and family eat at restaurants without worrying and don't get food poisoning?
Client: Maybe I'm overestimating the risk. They seem to trust that the food is safe. But isn't it better to avoid just to be on the safe side?
Therapist: Well, I agree with you that eating at restaurants is probably not as dangerous as you've been thinking, but it sounds like OCD is pushing you to eliminate all uncertainty – or to know the exact level of risk with complete certainty. But the truth is, that kind of certainty isn't possible – and even your friends and family don't have it. At the same time, it's not like the risk is 50:50. It seems low enough that people around you eat out without giving it much thought, and they haven't had issues like food poisoning. More importantly, what are the pros and cons of always trying to eliminate all risk? How has that interfered with your quality of life? What if you could learn to be more comfortable with this kind of uncertainty the way that your friends and family are?

Intolerance of Uncertainty

Help the client understand how intolerance of uncertainty contributes to OCD

As we have discussed, an important function of avoidance and compulsive rituals is to try to attain certainty about obsessional fears. It is as if clients need complete reassurance that something is safe, otherwise they perceive it as dangerous. This is in contrast to people without OCD, who generally have the adaptive ability to *feel* certain despite the fact that absolute certainty is more or less an illusion. You can use the demonstration in Clinical Vignette 6 to illustrate this:

Clinical Vignette 6
Challenging Intolerance of Uncertainty

Therapist: Think about someone you love very much [who is not in the room]. Is this person alive right now?
Client: Of course. Why do you even ask?
Therapist: I'm interested in how you know they're alive *for sure*?
Client: This morning I talked with them.
Therapist: But that was a few hours ago. Isn't it possible that something terrible could have happened since then?
Client: I've never thought about it that way ... So, maybe I don't know for *certain* that they're alive. But I would bet that they are.
Therapist: Of course, you would ... and I would too! What if you could use that same reasoning when it comes to your obsessional fears?

Point out that it is impossible to be 100% certain in most situations, and thus the goal of ERP is to learn how to make room for everyday levels of uncertainty. Medical emergencies, after all, *can* occur at any time. Yet, in the vignette, the client based her judgment on a *probability* as opposed to a *guarantee* of safety. Next, discuss other reasonable "risks" that the client takes on a regular basis (e.g., driving to and from the therapy session, crossing the street) to demonstrate that the client knows how to properly manage everyday levels of uncertainty in many areas of life. To reduce OCD symptoms, however, the client must be willing to practice living with uncertainty about obsessional fears as well.

Intolerance of uncertainty underlies obsessional fears of events that might occur in the *distant future* or are "unknowable" (e.g., cancer from long-term exposure to pesticides, going to Hell, becoming a pedophile). Clients often argue that they "cannot take the chance" of the feared event coming true. Here, you can point out that they would benefit by developing an alternative, less threatening, interpretation of the experience of uncertainty (that could subsequently be tested out using exposure techniques). This is illustrated in Clinical Vignette 7 with a client whose obsessional fears concerned the possibility of developing schizophrenia:

Clinical Vignette 7
Managing Fears of Future Uncertain OCD-Related Events

Therapist: When the thought that you could develop schizophrenia shows up, how do you respond?
Client: Well, I can't take the chance that I might go crazy!
Therapist: OK; and where does that lead you?
Client: I get worried, so I ask everyone for reassurance.
Therapist: Got it. And if you apply the same strategy that you say you used when I asked you about your loved one being alive, what could you tell yourself about those thoughts that would help reduce OCD?
Client: That the thoughts *probably* do not mean I am developing schizophrenia.

Therapist: That's right; they're *probably* just "mental noise" even though we don't have a guarantee. And although you can't really be 100% sure, you would probably be better off accepting *some* uncertainty and seeing this uncertainty as manageable. I bet you could learn to do this even though it might seem frightening. Do you think it would be worth testing out whether you could tolerate reasonable uncertainty about developing schizophrenia?

Significance of Thoughts (Thought–Action Fusion)

The belief that merely *thinking* about taboo or other unwanted or "off-limit" topics (e.g., blasphemous, aggressive, or sexual thoughts) is equivalent to "immoral" behavior indicates the need for additional discussion regarding the universality of intrusive thoughts. Ask the client what they think of the fact that even virtuous, ethical, and kind people sometimes have similar unwanted thoughts. If a double standard is present, point this out and discuss alternative explanations. It might also be helpful to point out that trying to analyze or pin down the precise meaning of a thought is akin to trying to obtain certainty about matters that cannot really be known for certain (i.e., it is a mental ritual).

If the client believes that unwanted thoughts will cause or lead to the corresponding event, explore their ideas regarding the mechanism by which this could occur (e.g., "How do you think your thoughts of stabbing your baby will lead you to *commit this action*?" "How will thinking about your sister having a car accident *make it happen*?"). Inconsistencies with reasoning can then be explored through Socratic questioning to encourage the client to rethink such assumptions (e.g., "If thoughts lead to actions, how are people ever able to maintain control of themselves when they get angry?" "Can you recall a time when you thought of something and it didn't happen?").

If the client is concerned that such obsessions imply they are a dangerous or immoral person, the discussion can focus on the *kinds* of people who would and would not be upset by thoughts of violence, blasphemy, or sexuality. Unlike the client, someone intent on committing violence would not worry if they had thoughts about such behavior. A sexual predator, for example, would not be plagued by doubts about whether they looked at a child the wrong way. An atheist would not be concerned over sacrilegious images.

Some clients are afraid that they are "not bothered enough" by their intrusive unwanted thoughts, and use this as the basis for their fear. This, however, implies intolerance of uncertainty regarding "how bothered is one supposed to be?" and "how much distress is enough?" These are unanswerable questions best addressed by learning to accept such uncertainties.

Does the client have a history of behavior or thoughts consistent with these obsessions? (Probably not.) Thus, you might also point out that although one's history can be telling, it is still not a guarantee; and the client is better off learning to manage the acceptable degree of uncertainty associated with these fears. Moreover, you might challenge the client to find even one person who has never had an "immoral" thought. But does this imply that everyone is immoral? You can use the experiment described in Clinical Vignette 8 to further illustrate this point.

Clinical Vignette 8
Illustration of the Cognitive Model With Non-OCD-Relevant Situation

Therapist: (*Hands the client a paper weight and says*) I want to you think about throwing this paper weight through the window of my office. Just let yourself think about it for a while.
Client: Are you sure?
Therapist: Yes. In fact, why don't you cock your arm back as if you were about to throw it.
Client: (*skeptically*) All right; it's your window! (*Holds his arm up to throw, but never actually throws the paper weight.*)
Therapist: (*after about a minute*) So, what's going on? How come you haven't thrown the weight?
Client: Well, obviously, I don't want to break your window.
Therapist: But you've been *thinking* about it, right?
Client: Yes. I see what you're getting at.
Therapist: And what is that?
Client: I guess it takes more than just thinking about doing something to make me do it.
Therapist: Yeah, that seems right. And what other factors might influence your behavior?
Client: Well, it's the wrong thing to do, and you'd probably make me pay for it.
Therapist: So, you're saying that you can make these decisions for yourself and that thoughts by themselves don't just translate into acting on impulse. Do you see how this relates to your obsessional thoughts of stabbing people you love? Your thoughts don't decide your actions ... *you* do!

Need to Control Thoughts

The need to control thoughts follows from dysfunctional beliefs about the importance of thoughts

The need to control thoughts follows from the belief that intrusive thoughts are highly significant and threatening. However, if clients are unaware of how their attempts at thought control are futile, they might believe that since they cannot control their thoughts, something must be terribly wrong with them. One technique for demonstrating the futility of attempts to control unwanted thoughts is the following experiment:

Therapist: Let's try an experiment. I'd like you to try not to think of a pink elephant for 1 minute. You can think of anything else in the world except for a pink elephant. OK? Go.

How to demonstrate the futility of trying to suppress obsessional thoughts

Invariably, the client will think of pink elephants and agree that it is nearly impossible to fully suppress such thoughts. Next, ask the client to explain how this phenomenon applies to obsessional thoughts. Such a discussion should focus on how attempts to suppress obsessional thoughts lead to a vicious cycle of more obsessions, futile attempts to suppress them, and so on. In fact, it is likely even more difficult to suppress obsessional thoughts (compared with pink elephant thoughts) given how personally relevant they are and how meaningful clients interpret them to be. It is understandable that at a certain point the client would believe (incorrectly) there is something wrong with their mind since they cannot suppress their thoughts. Of course, suppression attempts are unnecessary since obsessional thoughts are not dangerous in the first place.

Perfection, Symmetry, Order, and Not Just Right Experiences

In addressing the need for symmetry and the need to eliminate *not just right experiences*, help the client recognize that striving for absolute perfection or symmetry is impractical and unnecessary. Encourage the client to identify situations unrelated to OCD where they tolerate and accept imperfection and asymmetry without distress (e.g., unevenly arranged items on a desk or slightly crooked pictures on a wall). This helps the client understand that they are capable of managing not just right feelings and can extend this acceptance to situations influenced by OCD.

Excessive focus on perfection and symmetry hinder progress in therapy, leading to avoidance of tasks if perfect alignment cannot be achieved (e.g., "If it's not perfectly symmetrical, I can't start or complete it"). To counteract this, guide the client to deliberately create or leave slight asymmetries in tasks and observe the outcomes. This experiment allows the client to confront and assess whether the anticipated negative consequences (e.g., distress that spirals out of control) actually materialize, helping them to gradually reduce their compulsion for symmetry.

Clinical Pearl

Capitalizing on Opportunities to Maximize Cognitive Change

A few examples of how cognitive therapy strategies can be informally applied at various points in ERP are:

- During exposure exercises (described in Section 4.1.7), help the client process their experience. Review evidence regarding their ability to manage anxiety and uncertainty that is gleaned by performing the exercise. Help the client articulate more realistic beliefs about the experiences of obsessional thoughts, anxiety, guilt, disgust, and uncertainty.
- When a client shows strong affect, ask about the thoughts and images leading to their emotional response *at that moment*. Using Socratic questioning, address dysfunctional beliefs and assumptions. Apply this to OCD as well as to unrelated issues that may arise (e.g., a romantic break-up).
- Point out and summarize changes in beliefs (e.g., "I can't handle not knowing for sure") during and after the completion of exposure exercises. Ask them questions such as, "What did you learn from this exercise" or "What surprised you?"
- If self-monitoring forms indicate continued ritualizing, help the client identify dysfunctional cognitions. For example, "What were you saying to yourself when you saw the fire engine and decided to go home to check whether the appliances were unplugged?" and "What were the short- and long-term consequences of your ritualizing?"

4.1.5 Using Acceptance-Based Strategies

Acceptance and commitment therapy (ACT; Hayes et al., 2011) is a form of CBT that helps individuals learn to make room for unwanted thoughts and feelings, while committing to actions that align with their values. Rather than trying to eliminate distress, ACT focuses on changing one's relationship to it. Accordingly, ACT can be applied in the treatment of OCD to help clients foster a willingness to experience their obsessional thoughts, uncertainty, and anxiety nonjudgmentally without trying to resist them (Twohig et al., 2024). As with cognitive therapy, we suggest that ACT techniques are best used to foster treatment engagement and help facilitate ERP, rather than on their own. That is, we recommend integrating ACT principles throughout treatment to help clients understand exposure therapy as a means of learning to respond flexibly in the presence of obsessions, anxiety, disgust, and uncertainty. It is also helpful in linking specific exposures to improvements in quality of life and pursuing things in life which the client values.

Although ACT is sometimes cast as a distinct approach from traditional forms of CBT, including ERP, it is actually highly consistent with the model of OCD we presented in Chapter 2. An important goal of both ACT and ERP is to broaden the client's engagement with feared stimuli and improve quality of life. ACT, however, focuses more explicitly on (a) fostering willingness to experience obsessional distress, (b) recognizing thoughts and feelings as neither right nor wrong (i.e., *cognitive defusion*), and (c) using treatment to move toward what one values in life. For more information about ACT, the reader is referred to Hayes et al. (2011).

Fostering Willingness

ACT techniques foster willingness to experience obsessional distress

Willingness, in this context, refers to being open to "experiencing your own experience" without trying to change, avoid, or escape it. The metaphors in this section can be discussed to help the client understand the goal of treatment as developing a healthier (more peaceful) relationship to OCD-related inner experiences.

Two Scales

Explain to the client that it is relatively easy to rate the intensity of distress from obsessions on a scale from 0 to 100, and that they likely recognize many triggers that increase distress, often leading to avoidance and rituals to try to keep this distress as low as possible. However, these distress-reduction strategies work only temporarily and are not successful in the long-term. Obsessions and anxiety are usually very difficult (if not impossible) to control. But there is another less noticeable scale that is more important to focus on, because it is easier to control: This is the *willingness scale* which also goes from 0 to 100, and represents how open the client is to experiencing obsessions, anxiety, and doubts without trying to change or avoid them. Initially, the client will have this scale set very low, as indicated by the compulsive use of avoidance and rituals to try to resist obsessional distress. The problem is that when willingness is low, obsessional distress will often be high, because this sort of distress only gets worse when it is resisted. That is, "if you don't want it, you'll have it," meaning that if the client is unwilling to have intrusive thoughts, then intrusive thoughts are something to obsess about. Ask the client what would happen if their willingness scale value was set closer to 100. If this were the case, obsessions, anxiety, and feelings of uncertainty would be free to move around, come and go, etc. In other words, the client would be changing their relationship to thoughts and feelings for the better and would not have to use avoidance and rituals to fight them anymore. In fact, the distress scale would become less important. Exposure practices help the client increase their willingness to experience discomfort, and you can check in with them during exposure practices to assess how willing they are to experience distress.

Unwelcome Guest at the Party

In this metaphor, the client imagines themself hosting a party. They have invited their entire neighborhood, but then realize that someone they do not like (the unwelcome guest) has shown up at their door. The unwelcome guest represents all of the situations, thoughts, and feelings associated with OCD, and the client spends their time guarding the door and trying to keep the guest from coming in and ruining the party. In doing so, however, they are missing out on all the fun of the party (which represents their life). Ask the client what it would be like to welcome the unwanted guest into the party and be willing to have them there, even though the client does not care for them and does not like that they showed up. The guest is hard to ignore, and it would be better if they went home – but at least the client is engaging in the party and talking to their friends instead of guarding the door and missing out. This could lead to discussions about being willing to have obsessional thoughts, anxiety, guilt, disgust, and feelings of uncertainty even though they are unpleasant. In fact, in time, the client might find that the guest is not so terrible after all, even if they can't be ignored altogether. ERP will create opportunities to practice "letting the unwelcome guest into the party."

Tug-of-War With a Monster

Set a scene in which the client is about to play tug-of-war with a very strong monster (which represents OCD-related inner experiences). The client is on one side of a large canyon, and the monster is on the other, each holding one end of a rope. The loser of this match will fall over the cliff and into the canyon. Discuss with the client what options they seem to have: They could (a) pull the monster over the cliff (which is unlikely given how big and strong the monster is), or (b) be pulled over the cliff by the monster. But then point out that there is a third option: to drop the rope and disengage from the fight. In this case, the monster would still be there, but the fight would be over. Not only that, when there is no fight, the client is able to focus on other important things in life. The goal of ERP is to practice dropping the rope and living life even though the monster (i.e., anxious feelings, negative thoughts) is still there on the other side of the canyon.

Defusing From Thoughts and Feelings

Defusion: seeing obsessions for what they really are, not what they say they are

People with OCD often give their thoughts, feelings, and body sensations a great deal of power, such as when they view certain internal experiences as objectively "good" (e.g., calmness, control) or "bad" (e.g., obsessions, anxiety, uncertainty). The following metaphors can be used to help shift away from judging OCD-related internal experiences in this way (e.g., as "dangerous," "immoral," etc.), and learn to step back and simply observe these thoughts and feelings. Put another way, the aim is to see obsessions and anxiety for what they really are (streams of words, passing sensations), not what they "say" they are (facts or dangers).

Passengers-on-the-Bus Metaphor

In this metaphor, the client is driving a bus (which represents progress toward what they value in life) with some rowdy passengers aboard. These passengers (which represent OCD-related inner experiences) are scary looking, and they are yelling nasty threats (e.g., about obsessions, feared consequences, etc.) and insisting that the driver take the bus in a certain direction. The driver (client) has struck a deal with these passengers: As long as they hide at the back of the bus and stop yelling nasty and threatening things, the client promises to drive the bus wherever these passengers wish. That situation, however, represents giving in to OCD and letting it control their life. One seeming alternative is for the driver to stop the bus and try to kick the passengers off. But the passengers are very strong, so this does not work. What is more, the driver has to stop the bus to fight with the passengers, so it is no longer moving forward toward the client's values. Most clients (drivers) have tried this and failed at various points. The best solution, therefore, is to continue driving the bus in the valued direction and recognize that the worst thing these passengers can do is come up to the front of the bus, look scary, and yell nasty and threatening things. Although they look scary, the passengers cannot force the driver to go places the driver does not choose to go.

Becoming the Chess Board

Begin this metaphor by describing a game of chess with its two opposing teams. Team A represents OCD-related inner experiences (anxiety, obsessions, fears, doubts, disgust, etc.), while Team B represents feelings of safety, reassurance, and being in control. The client is asked which team they would prefer to help win the game (mostly likely, they will choose Team B). But the therapist can point out that the two opposing teams are actually both within the client; so, as soon as the client chooses a side, they are fighting themselves and therefore can never win the game. The therapist can then ask how things would be different if the client were the *chess board*, instead of one of the teams. If the client is part of a team, fighting and winning the game is very important, but if they are the board, they are in *contact* with the pieces (noticing them and remaining aware of what they are doing), but the outcome of the game is not important anymore.

Moving Toward Values in Life

Improving quality of life is an important outcome of ERP. The point of the following exercise is to help clients realize that the hard work of treatment is worthwhile.

Moving-Through-a-Swamp Metaphor

Ask the client to think of OCD-related inner experiences, and the situations that trigger them, as being like a swamp with mud, thick vegetation, moving rivers, quicksand, foul smells, and even creepy animals. On the other side of the swamp is a better quality of life. The client can try to avoid going into the swamp and getting dirty, but then they are not heading toward the things that are important. When the client practices ERP, they are learning how to handle whatever comes up while moving forward through this swamp. Point out that the client is getting dirty for a reason – they are not just wallowing in the swamp; the point of ERP is not just to make the client feel uncomfortable, but to move closer to what they want to get out of life.

4.1.6 Planning for Exposure and Response Prevention

In ERP, a client's obsessive fears are seen as learned threat associations where certain objectively safe thoughts or situations (e.g., senseless thoughts of acting impolitely) have become linked with distress (e.g., "These are dangerous thoughts that will lead me to act rudely"). The goal of ERP is to create new, safety associations (e.g., it is safe to think about acting impolitely) and to maximize the likelihood that these safety associations will win out over the threat-based associations, by ensuring they are as durable and generalizable as possible. To do this, therapists help clients approach their feared thoughts or situations (exposure) without performing their usual rituals to neutralize the fear (response prevention). Over time, as clients address these fears and see that the dreaded outcomes either do not happen or are not as bad as they anticipated, they start to form new safety-based associations to compete with the older threat-based associations. They also start to see how resisting rituals and combating avoidance improves their quality of life, and they develop a sense of self-efficacy in their ability to tolerate distress and engage in a healthy way with their fears.

Setting Treatment Goals

Before beginning a course of ERP, it is helpful for the client to take some time to identify their goals for treatment. What do they want to be different 3 months from now in terms of how they relate to their obsessions? How do they want to manage their urges to engage in compulsive rituals differently? How do they want their quality of life to improve? Goals should be specific, measurable, and concrete so that clients and therapists can know when they have reached them. Therapists should also ensure that goals are realistic and achievable. For instance, watch out for goals like "eliminate my anxiety," which would not be possible (or even recommended). Record these goals on the *Goal Setting in ERP Worksheet* (see Appendix 4). Periodically throughout treatment (e.g., every 2–3 months), check in about the client's progress toward their goals.

Choosing Items for the Exposure List

Design an exposure list tailored to a client's feared cues

An exposure list is a collection of all of the fear-provoking thoughts, situations, and cues the client will approach during therapy. The therapist should help the client rate how distressing each item is expected to be. Traditionally, these items are ranked by distress level and addressed gradually, starting with less distressing items and moving to more distressing ones. However, research suggests that mixing up the order (e.g., randomly selecting items from different levels of fear) can be even more effective (e.g., Craske et al., 2014). This varied approach teaches clients they can handle different levels of anxiety, enhancing their safety learning as discussed further in the following sections.

External Cues

Informed by the functional assessment, and with the client's assistance, compose a list of between 10 and 20 situations and stimuli that evoke the client's obsessional fears. Record these situations on the *Exposure List* form (see Appendix 5). Suggestions for choosing suitable exposure items appear below. Examples of exposure lists appear in Chapter 5.

The guiding principle when deciding on exposure items is that these situations and stimuli should closely match the client's particular obsessional fears. Therefore, those with contamination fears might work with items such as floors, elevator buttons, toilets, shoes, door handles, bodily waste and secretions, using pesticides, hospitals, shaking hands with possibly "contaminated" people, etc. Items that serve as reminders of contaminants (e.g., a roll of toilet paper) might also be incorporated if such stimuli are avoided. Exposure for clients with fears of mistakes or harm (negligence) might involve leaving the stove on and going outside, locking the door in a "careless" way, completing assignments hastily, driving past pedestrians, or thinking of insults before sending emails to important people (for someone afraid of sending insulting messages by mistake). Individuals with fears of bad luck might engage with "unlucky" numbers (e.g., 13, 666) or words (e.g., "death"). Those with obsessions about violence would encounter items that trigger such thoughts, such as knives and news stories about violence. Those with obsessions with sexual or religious themes would work with items such as provocative images, written scenarios, or religious icons. Finally, for clients with concerns about symmetry and order, exposure would entail producing the kinds of imperfection, disorder, imbalance, etc. that the person tries to avoid. Details for how to conduct exposure to these various stimuli are provided in Section 4.1.7.

Choose exposure tasks that represent *ordinary levels of risk* within the confines of your (or an expert's) judgment. Situations or stimuli that evoke high levels of obsessional fear must be included on the exposure list in order for clients to maximally benefit from treatment. Failure to address items that trigger high levels of anxiety prevents the full extinction of obsessional fear and reinforces the mistaken idea that such situations (and high levels of distress or fear) should be avoided because they really are too dangerous. This leaves clients vulnerable to the return of obsessional fear.

It is not essential that every possible fear cue appear on the exposure list. Items should be detailed enough to advise the client and therapist of the nature of the exposure exercises (public bathrooms), yet leave open the option to vary the specific task(s) in accord with the client's specific fears and in different contexts (e.g., bathrooms at home, at the mall, in restaurants, etc.). This permits flexibility in developing exposures of varying degrees of difficulty, as needed (some of which might not be contrived until the particular exposure is begun). Clinical Vignette 9 illustrates how to select exposure items collaboratively with the client.

Clinical Vignette 9
Putting Together an Exposure List

Therapist: You said that you limit your driving because you are afraid of hitting pedestrians. So, it sounds like a good situation for you to practice for exposure would be driving through the mall parking lot on a weekend afternoon.

Client: Oh no, I couldn't do that! I'd be too afraid. Maybe I could do it on a weekday when there are fewer people around.

Therapist: Well, as you know, the point of exposure is to practice approaching situations where you feel afraid so you can learn that they are safer than you think and see that you can manage the anxious feelings better than you expected. So, suppose we *begin* with driving through the parking lot on a weekday so you can get some experience with that and see how it goes, and then we plan to come back on a weekend? We can also try this exposure during the nighttime to help you learn that it is reasonably safe at different times of the day; but avoiding the weekend altogether would not be a good choice.

Client: I know, but it's hard for me to do.

Therapist: I hear you. That's why I'm OK with us starting with a weekday. It will give you a chance to see that you can manage driving in a parking lot. Then, we can go from there. I have confidence in you!

Client: Thanks for understanding. That sounds like a good plan.

Internal Cues

Imaginal exposure provides a systematic way of repeating and prolonging practice with approaching intrusive obsessional thoughts, images, and urges that evoke anxiety. Scenes to be imagined are chosen from the list of obsessional thoughts and ideas of feared consequences generated during the functional assessment. Brief descriptions of these scenes are entered onto the *Exposure List* form as well (Appendix 5).

Imaginal exposure can be used in different ways, either alone or in combination with exposure to external cues. Clients can conjure up anxiety-evoking intrusive thoughts and images, such as distressing, graphic, vulgar, or sacrilegious images (e.g., descriptions of accidents involving loved ones) as well as thoughts of, and uncertainty regarding, the feared consequences of exposure without performing rituals. For example, a client with fears of causing house fires by mistake might leave the iron plugged in (situational exposure) and, after leaving home without checking, purposely imagine that they have caused a serious fire (imaginal exposure). Imaginal exposures are especially useful for feared consequences like this, that would obviously not be safe or ethical to confront in real life (e.g., purposely burning down one's home, hitting a pedestrian, or contracting a serious illness) as well as for explicitly targeting uncertainty in exposures (e.g., writing about how one will never know for sure if they will one day snap and stab someone).

Clinical Pearl

Targeting Feared Consequences With Exposure

The best exposures are those which allow the client to test (and disconfirm) their fears of disastrous consequences (e.g., "I will hit someone with my car"). However, in some instances, feared consequences pertain to disasters either in the distant future (e.g., I will develop cancer in 10 years because I was near pesticides) or that are simply unknowable (e.g., I caused strangers to get COVID when I took off my mask to eat during the flight) and are therefore not subject to immediate disconfirmation. In such cases, where the fear cannot be tested, exposure tasks can be designed with the aim of learning that uncertainty over obsessional fears is manageable. Specifically, the client can encounter the feared situation or image, and then test their ability to manage the associated uncertainty without resorting to rituals such as confession or reassurance seeking. Rather than trying to disconfirm whether something terrible will happen, the emphasis is on helping the client see they can manage without rituals for longer (e.g., a specified number of minutes or hours) than they predicted they could.

Rating Items on the Exposure List

How to use the SUDS scale

Once an initial list of items is generated, ask the client to assign a numerical rating of *subjective units of distress* (SUDS) for each item (i.e., "How anxious would you feel if you engaged with ______?"). The SUDS scale includes every number from 0 (*no distress*) to 100 (*maximal distress*), although it can be introduced using the anchors shown below:

- 0 SUDS = no distress (like you are asleep)
- 25 SUDS = minimal distress
- 50 SUDS = moderate distress
- 75 SUDS = high distress
- 100 SUDS = maximum distress (like you're tied to the railroad tracks and the train is coming around the bend)

Record the client's SUDS rating for each item on the *Exposure List* form. Some considerations for using the exposure list to generate a treatment plan are as follows:

- One might begin with moderately distressing items (e.g., 40 SUDS) and work gradually up to those that are most distressing. A limitation of this approach is that it implicitly teaches clients that higher levels of anxiety are more threatening or more difficult to manage than lower levels. This could be problematic if it reinforces the experience of anxiety as a fear stimulus. Additionally, it could lead clients to experience anticipatory anxiety for items at the top of the hierarchy.

- Another approach is to allow clients to select the order of exposures based on how much they interfere with functioning or based on their importance in the client's life (i.e., values). For example, an exposure to holding a steak knife might be conducted earlier in treatment even though it is perceived by the client to be more challenging than holding other sharp objects like scissors or a sharp pencil, because the client may want to get back to eating dinner with their family as soon as possible.
- A third option is to randomly choose exposure items from the list (e.g., using an online random number generator). This maximizes variability in provoked anxiety, which helps solidify learning. It also best helps prepare clients for everyday life outside the therapist's office, where feared stimuli may appear in any order, rather than gradually. Clients may further find that if they tackle items on the list that are more challenging sooner, it may have a *trickle down* effect in which less challenging items are now possible to tackle as well (thus, potentially shortening the course of treatment).
- For clients who have fears in multiple OCD symptom dimensions, it can be effective to focus on one domain for the first several sessions in order to allow the client to gain some mastery over that domain before moving onto a new one. That said, given the benefits of incorporating variability into exposure, you do not need to solely focus on one fear in its entirety before moving onto the next theme. So, for example, even if a client is continuing to work on exposure practice related to unwanted sexual thoughts at home, you could begin introducing in session exposures related to responsibility for harm once you and the client decide they are ready to add a new challenge.
- All exposure exercises should be repeated in different contexts (e.g., locations, unaccompanied, time of day).
- Over the course of treatment, the client should gradually take more of an active role in designing and implementing exposures, such that they are learning to become their own therapist.
- Items that were inadvertently omitted from the list can always be added after discussion with the client. In other words, the exposure list can be considered a living document.
- In most cases, each item is first introduced under the therapist's supervision and then practiced between sessions.

Response Prevention Plan

The response prevention plan typically involves gradually refraining from compulsions

Although the term "response prevention" engenders images of physically restraining clients from performing rituals, the procedure is fully voluntary. Optimally, the client completely abstains from all rituals and neutralizing behaviors beginning with the first exposure session. However, most clients will require a gradual approach to stopping their rituals. Key considerations when planning for response prevention appear next.

- Revisit the educational materials presented in earlier sections and emphasize the importance of *choosing not to ritualize.*
- Define the limits of response prevention and do not require that clients take more than acceptable risks. For example, if "no checking door locks" is a rule, allow for an exception when going on an extended vacation (e.g., one brief check). Keep in mind that some clients may find checking just once is a slippery slope, and not checking at all would be easier and more effective for them (e.g., closing and locking the door without checking at all that it is locked).
- Do not violate cultural or hygienic norms, or official safety precautions (e.g., as were provided during the COVID-19 pandemic). Clients with washing rituals, for example, should be allowed to shower and brush their teeth daily and to wash their hands after using the restroom or before eating (the Centers for Disease Control and Prevention [CDC] recommends 20 seconds). However, they should *reapproach* contaminants following these cleaning or washing behaviors. For example, a client with fears of dirty laundry might wash their hands but then touch their laundry that they believe to be contaminated immediately afterwards to maintain the "contaminated" feeling.
- Specify abstinence from *mini rituals* and subtle safety behaviors that might not initially be recognized (or reported) as OCD symptoms (e.g., subtle forms of reassurance seeking).
- If relatives or friends are involved in the client's rituals, encourage their help with response prevention.
- For clients who are initially unable to cease all rituals, consider a gradual approach in which instructions to stop rituals parallel exposure practices. For example, once a client engages with "trash can germs" during exposure, they would be asked to refrain from washing their hands after taking out the trash or throwing something away; but not necessarily after using the bathroom, if exposure to bathrooms has not yet been practiced (although they should reapproach trash cans after such a wash).
- In situations where the client cannot refrain from a ritual indefinitely, *response delay* can be used, in which the ritual is put off for a given period of time (and the client is challenged to see how long they can delay before performing the ritual). In order to see if this approach is effective, check in with clients to ensure that they are not simply counting the minutes until the response prevention clock is up, or repeatedly reassuring themselves that the task is safe because they are going to do the ritual eventually. Rather, encourage clients to practice willingness to experience anxiety during the response delay. Once the agreed-upon delay has passed, see if the client can delay the ritual even further (since sometimes they find the urge is not as strong once the time rolls around). Additionally, work on increasing the interval they are delaying over time, so that at some point they can remove the ritual entirely.
- In general, if we needed to choose between a client doing a more challenging exposure but with rituals, or a less challenging exposure with no

rituals, we would choose the latter in the spirit of fostering willingness to experience anxiety and building anxiety acceptance.

- Instruct clients to record lapses of response prevention on the *Self-Monitoring of OCD Rituals* form (Appendix 2). Lapses indicate trouble spots that require additional work.

Clinical Pearl

Enlisting a Designated Support Person

Some clients encounter difficulty conducting exposure and response prevention tasks independently (between sessions). It may be useful in such cases to designate a ***support person*** such as a close friend or relative who agrees to be available and assist with treatment (when called upon by the client). The support person should also meet with the therapist to receive instruction in how to help with treatment. The best support people are those who are able to be empathic yet firm. Individuals who are overinvolved in the client's symptoms, or who are overly critical or harsh, should be avoided. The support person is to report any adherence problems to the therapist. Importantly, when a support person becomes involved, the primary relationship remains between the therapist and client (e.g., no "secrets" shared by the support person would be kept from the client).

Some typical response prevention rules for common presentations of OCD are as follows:

Decontamination Rituals

Ideas for implementing response prevention for common compulsive rituals

Clients are asked not to use cleaning agents such as hand sanitizers or wet wipes on their body. Creams, makeup, and deodorants are allowed as long as they are not used to reduce contamination fears. One daily 10-minute shower is permitted, but ritualistic washing of specific body parts is not allowed (e.g., washing body parts in a certain order or a certain number of times; unless medical conditions necessitate such cleansing). Handwashing is permitted only after using the restroom, before eating, or if hands are visibly soiled (e.g., after gardening) and should be restricted to the CDC recommended 20 seconds. Following showering or handwashing, the client is asked to recontaminate with items from earlier exposures.

Checking, Counting, Arranging, and Repeating Rituals

The client is asked not to engage in any repetitive behaviors. For example, only *one* brief glance in the rearview mirror when driving, *one* quick check of the door when leaving the home, *one* rapid proof for errors when completing paperwork or sending electronic messages, etc. Checking and counting are not allowed for items normally not checked (e.g., whether appliances are plugged in) or counted (e.g., steps). Counting and checking rituals may be foiled by counting incorrectly, checking incompletely, or reminding oneself that they are not 100% certain of the outcome of the check. Actions repeated because of the presence of "bad thoughts" (e.g., going back and forth through a doorway until blasphemous thoughts are successfully suppressed) are not to be repeated. Rearranging items that appear imperfect is not allowed.

It can be helpful to share with clients that research suggests that the more people go back and check something, the *less* confidence they have in their own memory (e.g., Jondani et al., 2023). Clients are often surprised to hear this information, and sometimes just knowing the counterproductive nature of checking can facilitate response prevention.

Reassurance-Seeking Rituals

Compulsive reassurance seeking from family members, "experts" (e.g., priests, doctors), or from the therapist, is not permitted. It is helpful to set the stage early in treatment when conceptualizing (with the client's input) that these behaviors seem to reduce anxiety and uncertainty in the moment (when the client feels relief upon being reassured), they ultimately reinforce doubt and increase the urge to seek reassurance in the long run. Discuss with clients the difference between asking a question to legitimately gather new information and asking a question when the answer is already known, in order to reduce anxiety (which is a reassurance-seeking ritual). Be prepared that clients will likely seek reassurance from you at some point. When this happens, acknowledge their distress and desire for certainty, explain that answering the question would only reinforce OCD, and invite them to practice making room for uncertainty – in most cases, clients agree to give this a try. It can also be useful to educate others (e.g., family, friends) from whom the client habitually seeks reassurance, about the importance of refraining from answering these types of questions during treatment. Suggest that they respond in a supportive way. For example, a family member might say, "It sounds like you're having trouble with needing reassurance. I'm sorry but I can't answer that question because I agreed to help you with treatment. I know you're strong and can get through this without reassurance. What else could I do to help you manage your discomfort?"

Mental Rituals

Arranging response prevention for *mental rituals* can be challenging because mental rituals are not easily observable like most other compulsions. Clients might first need to learn to recognize the difference between their obsessions and their mental rituals (which can be a focus of the educational component of treatment described in Section 4.1.3). Response prevention includes refraining from mental strategies for canceling (neutralizing) or "putting right" unacceptable thoughts. Ritualized praying (i.e., used to deal with obsessional fear) is also prohibited, although healthy faithful prayer is allowed. If mental rituals cannot be easily stopped, suggest that the client (a) think of an *upsetting* thought instead or (b) perform the mental ritual incorrectly. For example, if the ritual is to mentally reassure oneself by reviewing events (e.g., to be sure one did not say racial slurs), the review should be purposely foiled (e.g., "I can't be sure if I'm remembering everything exactly the way it happened").

Mindfulness techniques can also be helpful for clients with mental rituals to learn flexible strategies for shifting their attention (e.g., catching themself when their mind gets caught up in obsessive thoughts and bringing it back to the present moment without engaging in mental rituals) and instead placing their focus on goals, values, or tasks at hand. In other words, these skills can be useful for helping clients "get out of their head" and return to their life. There are many mindfulness apps for smartphones that can be incorporated into treatment of OCD. Some commonly used apps include Headspace, Calm, Ten Percent Happier, and Buddhify.

Agreeing on the Treatment Plan

Before exposure begins, the client and therapist both agree to adhere to the treatment plan. Review the following points before moving on:

The client and therapist must agree on the treatment plan before ERP begins

- Beginning with the next session, the client will practice exposures by approaching the situations and thoughts on the exposure list as planned--both during sessions with therapist's supervision and coaching, and independently between sessions.
- The client will also practice refraining from rituals as planned, and let the therapist know if there are problems with resisting the urges.
- If an urge cannot be resisted, the ritual should be recorded on the *Self-Monitoring of OCD Rituals* form (see Appendix 2), and the client should reapproach the situation or thought which evoked the ritual.
- Daily self-guided exposure tasks will be assigned for practice between sessions. These tasks may be practiced alone or with the supervision of a designated support person but should be practiced in varied settings and contexts to be maximally effective.
- The client should expect to feel anxious when first addressing each new exposure situation, and understand that although challenging in the beginning, things will get easier with repeated practice. However, make sure clients understand that a primary goal of exposure is fostering anxiety acceptance, so that if fear reduction in a given exposure session does not occur, clients do not view this exercise as a failure. It is important to frame the exposure in such a way that clients leave feeling empowered rather than discouraged.
- The therapist will not force the client into doing exposure tasks but will *encourage* or *challenge* the client to choose exposure instead of avoidance.
- The therapist will assume the role of a coach who provides instruction and support throughout treatment. This means encouraging the client to approach their fears and *work through* the distress, rather than making the distress go away.
- Treatment should not proceed until the client agrees to this treatment plan and any questions and concerns are addressed.

4.1.7 Implementing Exposure and Response Prevention

This section describes how to conduct exposure therapy for OCD. The basic format of each exposure session is outlined in Table 7. The primary goal of these sessions is for the client to approach and engage with the predetermined fear cue(s) without performing rituals. In some exposure sessions, distress levels will decline over time, while in others, this habituation may not occur. Because the goal is to learn anxiety acceptance, each exposure can continue until either the distress level (and compulsive urges) dissipates on its own, or the client is able to manage what distress is present. Accordingly, there is no strict rule about the duration of each exposure session. Most exposures can be conducted within the framework of the typical 50- to 60-minute outpatient appointment.

Table 7
Components of Exposure Sessions

Procedure	Approximate time
Checking in, reviewing exposure practice homework, and reviewing self-monitoring forms	10–15 minutes
Conducting the in-session exposure exercise	30–35 minutes
Agreeing on homework practice	5 minutes
Planning for the next session's exposure	5 minutes

Clinical Pearl
Goals for Early Exposure Sessions

To strengthen the client's trust and participation in exposure therapy, it is important to appear hopeful and confident. Showing an understanding of the client's OCD symptoms, being up front when discussing the treatment procedures, and taking seriously the client's input help strengthen the client's conviction in the treatment program.
During initial exposure sessions, help the client develop good *work habits* for performing these tasks by attending to (and shaping) their behavior. Many will have never tried this type of exercise before or might have tried it and stopped because it provoked high levels of distress. Additionally, exposure exercises typically represent the exact *opposite* of what clients have been doing to manage their OCD. Explain why evoking distress is a central part of exposure – it helps the client learn that anxiety, uncertainty, guilt, disgust, etc. are safe, manageable, and time limited. Be democratic (as opposed to autocratic) and show sensitivity to help the client view you as an advocate, rather than a drill sergeant!

Checking Homework and Reviewing Self-Monitoring Forms

Reinforce the importance of homework by checking the client's forms at the start of each session

Each exposure session begins with a general check-in and review of homework assignments. All forms are reviewed (although you may choose to discuss only 1 or 2 exposure practices in detail in the interest of time) and the client provides a qualitative report of the work they completed between sessions. Follow up on the exposure assignments you gave the client in the previous session and review self-monitoring forms of OCD rituals to reinforce the importance of working hard between sessions. This will also help you determine whether all instructions have been followed correctly. Use praise to reinforce successful completion (or sufficient effort toward completing) assigned tasks. Be sure to process what the client has learned from completing each assignment. When assignments are not completed as instructed, troubleshoot and, if necessary, complete the homework in that day's session before moving on (e.g., complete the self-monitoring of rituals form together, recalling rituals conducted that previous morning).

Introducing the Exposure Task

How to introduce the exposure task and response prevention plan

Begin by describing the specifics of the planned exposure task, including how the feared stimulus will be approached, and what kinds of distress-reduction behaviors (e.g., rituals) are to be resisted during and after the exercise. Then, help the client identify feared consequences of performing the exposure task. Some will articulate short-term consequences that can easily be tested during exposure, such as whether thinking racial slurs will lead to blurting them out loud, or whether leaving an appliance plugged in while out of the house will result in a fire. Others will fear long-term or unknowable consequences, such as gradually losing their intellectual abilities or causing bad luck to a loved one not in the room. Yet even these concerns have a short-term fear component – the immediate fear involves not knowing for sure whether the long-term consequences will occur or whether they can manage the distress, guilt, disgust, or "not just right" feelings associated with the exercise (i.e., intolerance of uncertainty). Thus, exposure can be used to help the client discover that such uncertainty is in fact manageable (i.e., not threatening enough to warrant avoidance or rituals).

Accordingly, when fears of long-term consequences are present, help the client identify shorter-term feared consequences that can be tested within the exposure session, such as "I won't be able to handle the uncertainty for more than a few minutes," "The anxiety will be too much for me to take and I will have to do a ritual," and "I won't be able to tolerate feeling 'not just right' for very long." Exposures to the possibility of these feared outcomes will test the client's beliefs about how long they can put up with distress without escaping by ritualizing. Ask the client for an estimate of how long they expect to be able to continue the exposure and endure the anxiety and uncertainty without ritualizing.

To give the client an idea of how the exercise is to proceed, review the *Guidelines for Conducting Exposure* handout (see Appendix 6) before beginning the first exposure. A brief description of the exercise, the feared consequences, and an initial SUDS rating should be entered on the *Exposure Practice Form* (see Appendix 7), which is used to keep track of progress during each exercise.

A typical introduction to an exposure task is as follows:

Therapist: At the end of our last meeting, we agreed that the exposure task for today would be for you to practice writing words you've been avoiding, such as "sin" and "demon." So, how about if you practice writing these words – and perhaps others – over and over on this pad of paper. I also want you to allow yourself to think about any distressing thoughts that may come to mind, such as the blasphemous images you are bothered by. Your job is to practice not "canceling out" these thoughts, or using prayer or confession rituals to make you feel less distressed. Instead, we're going to work on just making room in your mind for these kinds of upsetting thoughts. I know this is going to produce anxiety for you, but doing this exposure will help teach you that you can allow those thoughts to be there without trying to control them. You might even see that your distress subsides when you don't try to fight the thoughts so much. This exercise will also help you gain a sense of mastery over your fear. We will be keeping track of your anxiety level (SUDS) during the exposure by asking you to rate it every 5 minutes so you can see that you can handle these feelings. So, have in mind a number between 1 and 100 to give me. Any questions? Are you ready?

Conducting Exposure Exercises

How to conduct exposure exercises for common OCD symptoms

The aim of each exposure is to provide opportunities for the client to develop new safety-based associations with feared stimuli (both external situations and feelings such as anxiety and uncertainty themselves). To maximize this learning, conduct exposures so that they disconfirm the client's fear-based expectancies about obsessional stimuli as written on the *Exposure Practice Form* (Appendix 7; e.g., "I will start throwing up," "I won't be able to tolerate not knowing if God is upset with me for more than a few minutes"). In some instances, this will involve learning that feared stimuli are acceptably safe (i.e., the feared outcome is not as likely or as severe as was predicted). In others, it will involve learning that feelings of distress, fear, disgust, guilt, anxiety, and/or uncertainty are safe and manageable. Accordingly, exposure concludes when client's expectations of the danger or intolerability of feared stimuli have been contradicted. Learning focuses on whether the expected negative outcome occurred or was as "awful" as expected (i.e., was it more *manageable* than anticipated). In some cases, this will require that exposures be prolonged and repeated more than once.

A suggested strategy for enhancing extinction is to combine *multiple fear cues* during exposure sessions. For example, if a client's obsessional fear of harming loved ones is evoked by knives and by stories about serial killers, they might read stories about serial killers while handling knives in the presence of loved ones (note that these exposures – being in the presence of loved ones, handling knives, and reading about killers – would optimally first be conducted separately prior to being combined).

At regular intervals during the exposure, ask the client to rate their distress level (and perhaps their urge to ritualize), and record these ratings on the *Exposure Practice Form*. Research suggests that asking clients to *put their feelings into words* and verbalize them out loud helps consolidate learning during exposure (e.g., Craske et al., 2014). We therefore encourage therapists to ask questions such as "How are you feeling now?" and "What are you telling yourself about doing this exposure?" and record the answers (e.g., "I'm feeling very scared that I've caused an accident and I want to go back and check") on the *Exposure Practice Form*.

While it is important to maintain a general *attentional focus* on the exposure task, the conversation may occasionally drift off topic. When this occurs naturally, you can point out that the client is able to have a casual conversation even while encountering a feared stimulus and experiencing anxiety or uncertainty. This helps consolidate learning about their ability to tolerate the experience. Note that this situation is different from purposeful distraction from the exposure task, which is counterindicated. Accordingly, therapists should double check with clients that they are not deliberately steering the conversation in a different direction for this purpose.

When the exposure is complete, help to further *consolidate* what has been learned by asking the client to articulate what they discovered during the experience. Did their fears come true? Were anxiety and uncertainty truly unbearable? Did they manage disgust, guilt, or "not just right" feelings better than they thought? What surprised the client about doing the exposure – did it turn out to be easier than they expected? The answers to these types of questions can be discussed in the context of the client's initial (and now disconfirmed) expectations about the difficulty of the exposure. Help the client recognize that they can cope better than predicted with obsessional thoughts, anxiety, or uncertainty about feared consequences. To provide an overview of how response prevention tied to the feared exposure stimulus can then be continued between sessions, review the *Guidelines for Conducting Response Prevention* handout (see Appendix 9).

The next sections present detailed guidance for conducting situational and imaginal exposures for common presentations of OCD.

Contamination Fears

Begin by encouraging the client to touch the feared contaminant. If necessary, during early exposures, you might model this by touching the stimulus yourself. The client must *fully* engage with the feared stimulus – briefly touching it with fingertips does not count! It is important for the client to feel thoroughly contaminated and vulnerable to feared consequences, otherwise the threat-based prediction cannot be fully tested and disconfirmed.

Clinical Vignette 10 illustrates exposure to "contaminated" mail from the client's mailbox. The client fears that her mail carrier has contracted the COVID-19 virus and will pass it along to the client through contact with her mail. Note how the therapist structures the exposure to disconfirm the client's expectations about how long she can manage touching the envelopes. Also, note that there was no discussion of the inaccurate beliefs about how COVID-19 spreads. This was discussed during an earlier session that incorporated informal cognitive therapy, but the client is also learning – through direct experience during exposure – that these beliefs are not accurate.

Clinical Vignette 10

Example of an Exposure Exercise With Contamination Fears

Therapist: How about if we start with you touching the envelope with your whole hand.

Client: (hesitates) ...OK. (puts hand on the envelope) There.

Therapist: Good job. So, how do you feel right now?

Client: I'm scared that I'm going to get COVID from touching this envelope. I really think my mail carrier has COVID and doesn't take the right precautions to keep from spreading it. I'm not sure how long I can stand doing this.

Therapist: You're doing great. It's OK to feel anxious – remember the "bring it on" attitude! Anxiety is the raw material of change. It's worth feeling anxious now so that you can learn how to handle feelings of contamination and anxiety in the future. You predicted that you could touch the envelope for 5 minutes before you would absolutely have to wash your hands. Let's see if you can surprise yourself. What is your SUDS rating?

Client: About 80 [therapist records this on the form].

Therapist: How strong is your urge to wash your hands?

Client: Pretty strong. Like 85%.

Therapist: You're doing great. Keep your hand on the envelope.

5 minutes later...

Therapist: So, it's been 5 minutes , and you're still touching the envelope. What do you make of that?

Client: I'm surprised I could do it. I thought I'd have to run to the bathroom to wash.

Therapist: Good for you! How long do you think you could keep touching it now?

Client: I think I could do it for the rest of the session. I'm pretty confident even though my SUDS is still at 65. It doesn't seem to be so terrible once I just make myself do it.

Amplifying refers to deliberately intensifying an exposure in order to address a particular aspect of avoidance and to further test the client's expectations. For contamination exposures, this usually means spreading feared contaminants to items or body parts the client tries to avoid tainting (e.g., toothbrush, wallet, face, hair, mouth). As an example, the client in Clinical Vignette 10 was instructed to put the envelope in her lap and to touch it to her arms, legs, and face. This was repeated every 5 to 10 minutes varying areas of the body that were touched. For instance, she touched the envelope to her purse (inside and out), hair, and jacket for longer than she thought she could.

Look for subtle avoidance and rituals such as wiping off germs, opening doors with one's feet, and other curious maneuvers that most people do not do. Clients who appear to "space out" during exposure can be asked whether they are engaging in purposeful distraction or other strategies such as praying and analyzing the chances of getting sick. These rituals might be so habitual that they occur without the client's awareness. Therefore, try to bring them to the client's attention whenever they are observed.

The importance of matching the exposure to the client's obsessional fear cannot be overstated. Clients fearful of "spreading" contamination to other people should practice shaking hands with others. Those fearful of "floor germs" can conduct entire sessions seated on the floor (in a public bathroom, for example). For those concerned with bodily waste and fluids, we supervise direct encounters with such substances (or situations in which the substances *might* be present). Examples include, putting a drop of urine on the hand, deliberately stepping in dog poop and wiping it off with a tissue, and handling dirty towels found in the gym locker room (fear of sweat).

Obsessional Doubts of Harm and Negligence

There are a few complexities to be aware of when carrying out exposure for obsessions about mistakes and harm. First, it is important to make sure that the client does not transfer their feelings of responsibility onto the therapist. For example, during an exposure to writing emails, a client might notice that their therapist is watching closely, and this might foil the exposure task (e.g., "My therapist would never let me send an inappropriate email"). Second, many situational exposures for harming obsessions will be compromised if they are prolonged or repeated during the same session. For example, plugging in the iron or turning on the stove can only be done once during a single session because repeating these exercises is inherently a check that no fire has started. Accordingly, when performing these types of exposures with clients, take precautions to ensure that no de facto reassurance seeking occurs that would invalidate the exposure. For instance, ask the client if your mere presence is reassuring to the point that it makes the exposure easier; if so, have the client perform actions once on their own and then promptly leave the premises without checking. The exposure can then be prolonged using imaginal exposure to uncertainty about whether the feared consequences have (or will) occurred (e.g., the email might contain racial slurs, the house could be burning down). In these types of exposure, the client will test beliefs about their ability to manage uncertainty about these feared consequences for certain lengths of time ("I couldn't think about a fire without checking the house for more than an hour").

Exposure for harming, injury, and mistake obsessions can be complex

Some examples of exposure assignments for clients with harming obsessions and checking rituals are as follows: A client who fears hitting pedestrians can perform driving exposures without checking the roadside or mirror. Someone fearful of causing a fire or a burglary can practice carelessly turning off lights and appliances, or closing and locking doors, without checking. A client with fears of stabbing others can use knives and pins around other people. Someone with fears of cursing or insulting others can practice writing and saying curse words (see Section 4.6.2 for specific guidance regarding exposure to racial slurs).

When the feared act of commission or omission presents a very low risk of harm, exposure can involve deliberately carrying out such behaviors. A few examples are as follows: A client who fears that failing to warn others of glass on the floor will result in someone being injured can purposely place pieces of glass on the floor of a crowded area, refrain from warning people, and then practice imaginal exposure to the possibility that they caused injury. Someone fearful of starting a fire can intentionally leave appliances (even the stove) on and unattended for an acceptable period of time. A client who fears miswriting an address on an envelope can purposely misspell the addressee's name, street, or city. Someone afraid of numbers such as 13 or 666 can deliberately write these numbers on their hand or on pictures of people they would not want to "curse."

As mentioned previously, imaginal exposure should be integrated with situational exposure when clients report feared consequences of not checking. For example, a client with obsessional fears of leaving confidential information in plain view at work first completed a situational exposure involving handling confidential files, putting them away while distracted with music (he feared this would make him more likely to make such a mistake), and leaving for home without checking. Once he arrived home, he performed imaginal exposure to obsessional thoughts of mistakenly leaving files in plain sight, being caught and fired, and then being sued. The therapist introduced the imaginal exposure using the *Guidelines for Conducting Imaginal Exposure* (Appendix 8) as described in Clinical Vignette 11.

Clinical Vignette 11
Introducing an Imaginal Exposure

You said that when obsessional doubts of violating confidentiality come to mind, you often return to work to make sure you haven't left any confidential materials out on your desk – but you never find that you've actually made any of the mistakes you obsess over. It's just that this obsessional thought bullies you into the checking rituals to reduce your feeling of uncertainty and doubt. To help you learn a new agenda for responding to these obsessional doubts and urges to check, let's practice deliberately thinking the obsessional doubts; but instead of checking, your job is to allow the doubt and uncertainty to remain in your mind. You're going to practice making space for it and just notice these thoughts and feelings while you go about your routine. By doing this exercise repeatedly, you will see that you are able to manage these doubts better than you thought, even if you don't go back and check or try to mentally review your activities to reassure yourself. The goal is for you to learn that you can live your life and do what you need to do at home even if these obsessional doubts show up.
So, for this imaginal exposure, I will ask you to write a script in which you describe what you're afraid would happen if your worst fears come true. We will then make a recording of this script on your phone so you can listen to it over and over to bring on your anxiety and uncertainty. Every 5 minutes you can give your SUDS rating to track your anxiety level. Your job will be to lean into the doubts and uncertainty so you can learn that these feelings don't have to push you around into wasting your time checking or seeking reassurance.

The client then wrote a description of his feared consequences of leaving confidential materials on his desk and failing to check. The description was edited with the therapist to ensure that it contained elements that the client experienced as most distressing, such as his irresponsibility for the breach of confidentiality and the idea that he *should* have checked more carefully. The script was then recorded using a smartphone app so that the client could replay it and visualize the scene while engaging in activities at home, demonstrating that he could operate with the distress and uncertainty for longer than he predicted he could. By doing this, he learned that he could manage the obsessional distress. One thing to keep in mind with imaginal exposures is that they are sometimes more challenging than clients expect because clients are addressing their worst fears head on (especially when following the aforementioned guidelines to maximize their effectiveness).

Unacceptable Obsessional Thoughts

ERP for unacceptable thoughts involves exposure to external cues that trigger these obsessions, as well as imaginal exposure to obsessional thoughts and images themselves. Such exposures are repeated in multiple contexts to generalize learning. The example in Clinical Vignette 12 illustrates how to conduct an exposure session for a client with repugnant obsessional thoughts of stabbing someone.

Use imaginal exposure for repugnant obsessional thoughts

Clinical Vignette 12

Introducing an Exposure Exercise for Unacceptable Obsessional Thoughts

Today's exposure practice will help you become better at managing your unwanted thoughts about stabbing people and the distress that comes with these thoughts. We will start by writing a description of the obsessional thoughts, which we will record, and you will practice listening to it. You will also practice holding sharp objects, like a knife. Remember that we are working on not trying to fight or control these thoughts, so it will be important that you don't make any attempt to suppress, remove, or neutralize them. If you do feel yourself trying to remove the thought, let me know so I can help you remain engaged in the exposure. The goal of this exercise is not to make the thoughts go away, but to give you the opportunity to let your mind "go there" and learn to relate to these kinds of thoughts in a healthier way. I will keep track of your SUDS during the exercise.

The client was first helped to write a script of her obsessional thoughts. After editing with the therapist (to highlight the most distressing aspects, such as the idea of attacking someone by surprise), the final version, which the client audio recorded, was as follows:

Sharp objects can be dangerous. I could use them to stab people, which would badly hurt or kill them. When I use knives, I often think of stabbing innocent people and people that I especially care about, like my husband, Shawn. If I attacked someone by surprise, I could do a lot of damage with just a few thrusts of a knife in the right place, such as their neck, eyes, chest, stomach, or genitals. If a person is taken by surprise, they would not be ready to defend themselves and they would die of their stab wounds that I inflicted.

I could stab Shawn while he was sleeping. He would be unaware that I was doing it until the knife pierced his skin and entered his body. He might wake up in terror and try to fight off my stabbing, but he would lose so much blood that he wouldn't be able to fight me off. I could easily kill him by stabbing him in his sleep and would be unable to defend himself. There would be blood everywhere and he would be screaming from all the pain. If I stabbed him in the right place, I'd damage his vital organs and he would die.

The client predicted that she could only tolerate having this thought for 10 minutes without neutralizing because her distress would be "too high." So, exposure involved testing this out. After she was able to confront the thought for over 20 minutes with her SUDS at 90, the therapist helped her consolidate what she had learned so far – that she could remain engaged with the obsession and feelings of anxiety more than she thought she could. At that point, with her SUDS decreasing only to 75, the therapist gave the client a large butcher knife and asked her to hold it while listening to the recording. After an initial increase in SUDS back to 90, she was able to remain in the exposure without neutralizing for another 20 minutes. At that point (after receiving consent from the client), the therapist brought an office coworker into the room (who had volunteered to help with treatment). The recording was turned off, and the client was asked to hold the knife while talking with this confederate. Then, the confederate sat at a computer terminal while the client held the knife to the confederate's back and elicited stabbing thoughts. Finally, this exercise was continued with the therapist out of the room but checking in every 5 minutes to obtain a SUDS rating. The exposure was ended after 60 minutes, and the client and therapist discussed what had been learned in terms of acceptance of obsessions and anxiety. The client's SUDS were 70 when the exposure was ended, but she was confident that she could tolerate the anxiety.

Incompleteness Symptoms

Clients with incompleteness OCD symptoms may or may not articulate fears of harm. When the sense of inexactness, imperfection, or asymmetry does evoke obsessional fears of responsibility for disasters (e.g., "Dad will die if I do not put on my clothes the 'correct' way"), exposure to external cues should be conducted, accompanied by imaginal exposure to the feared consequences (as with harming obsessions). Remind clients to refrain from rituals such as ordering and arranging, checking and repeating, and reassurance seeking. One client who worried that stepping on sidewalk cracks would cause harm to his parents purposely stepped on cracks and confronted thoughts of his parents being injured because of this. Another feared bad luck from odd numbers and therefore practiced facing them wherever possible by purchasing items that cost $7.99, and choosing to be 9th in line. He also practiced wishing for bad luck to occur as a result of his confrontation with odd numbers.

When the client is mostly concerned that "not-just-right experiences" will persist indefinitely or spiral out of control unless rituals are performed, exposure aims to change beliefs about one's ability to tolerate these uncomfortable feelings while they are present. With prolonged and repeated exposure to the "imperfection," the client learns that the distress associated with these feelings is manageable, thereby rendering ordering rituals unnecessary.

Clinical Pearl

Integrating Cognitive Therapy With Exposure

On their own, well-formulated and well-conducted exposure exercises help the client develop more realistic estimates of the probability and severity of feared consequences. The client's ability to exceed their expectations of what they can handle also helps to modify maladaptive beliefs that anxiety, uncertainty, and other negative feelings that accompany obsessions are intolerable or will persist indefinitely. Cognitive therapy techniques can also be used at various points during exposure sessions to augment these cognitive changes – and preliminary research indicates that outcomes are comparable regardless of the timing of these cognitive strategies (Buchholz et al., 2022):

- *When initiating an exposure task*, cognitive techniques can be used to identify mistaken cognitions (e.g., "Thinking about harm is the same as causing harm") and feared consequences (e.g., "I will be responsible for a terrible accident") that can be tested during exposure.
- *During exposures*, cognitive techniques can be used to promote adaptive beliefs and responses to obsessional fear (e.g., "Even if something happens, it's not my fault").
- *After an exposure exercise*, Socratic discussion is used to help the client review the outcome of the exercise, examine evidence for and against the catastrophic beliefs, and develop more realistic beliefs about obsessional stimuli. Ask clients what they expect will happen the next time they confront the same feared stimuli; ideally these expectancies will have changed to be more benign when compared to the start of the exercise.

Prescribing Homework Practice

At the completion of each in-session exposure, assign practices for each day between sessions. Homework includes exposure, refraining from rituals and neutralizing, and continual self-monitoring of rituals that cannot be resisted. Consider the following points when designing homework assignments:

- Assign repetitions and variations of the in-session situational and imaginal exposure exercises.
- The more the client practices exposure to the same (or similar) stimulus under different conditions and in different situations, the better.
- Provide copies of the *Exposure Practice Form* to be completed during each homework assignment (Appendix 7). Specify the details of each assignment and be sure the client knows how to complete the form properly.
- Suggest that the client regularly review the *Guidelines for Conducting Exposure*, the *Guidelines for Conducting Imaginal Exposure*, and *Guidelines for Conducting Response Prevention* handouts (Appendix 6, Appendix 8, and Appendix 9).
- Reinforce the importance of homework by beginning each session with a check of the previously assigned work.

Planning for the Next Session

Conclude each session by reviewing progress and discussing plans for the next session's exposure

At the end of each session, the therapist should review the client's progress and discuss the task scheduled for the next session. If items need to be brought from the client's home (or from elsewhere), or if the session must take place out of the office, this should be arranged.

Conducting Exposure to Very Distressing Stimuli

Although clients will likely be hesitant to attempt exposure to stimuli that provoke a great deal of anxiety and fear, learning that even high levels of distress are manageable is important for long-term improvement. Accordingly, try to strike a balance between encouraging clients to push themselves (i.e., a "bring it on" attitude) and letting them decide when they are ready. Consider that procrastination on the client's part might be a form of avoidance. In fact, clients might find that the anticipatory anxiety about these most distressing stimuli may be worse than completing the exercise itself, indicating the benefits of tackling these exposures sooner rather than later. It can be helpful to review educational materials about the nature of anxiety (e.g., the fight-or-flight response is a normal and adaptive process that is not dangerous). It is important to use such exposures to target the client's beliefs about their ability to manage anxiety along with beliefs about feared consequences. Be sure to allow time to repeat these exposures in varied contexts, since fear extinction is most complete and long-lasting when feared stimuli are confronted in a variety of circumstances, as opposed to only in the therapist's office.

Clinical Pearl
Helping Clients Confront Their Greatest Fears

You can use the following tactics to help clients who are having difficulty attempting the most difficult exposures:

- Empathize with the discomfort.
- Model the task prior to instructing the client to engage.
- Use intermediate exposures that are of greater difficulty than those already conducted, but not as difficult as the planned task (the client must agree that the intermediate step serves to facilitate eventual exposure with the more difficult item).
- Use Socratic dialog to help the client challenge maladaptive beliefs about the dangerousness and tolerability of anxiety.
- Review evidence collected during previous exposures.
- Discuss the importance of learning to take acceptable risks.
- Revisit the importance of learning to tolerate uncertainty.
- Refer to ACT metaphors as necessary.
- Ask clients to describe the ways in which conducting this exposure would move them closer to their values and/or improve their quality of life.
- Remind clients that the more work (and anxiety) they invest in this treatment, the more they'll get out of it in the long run.

With the strategies above, therapists should keep in mind that spending extra time discussing an exposure can prolong anticipatory distress. Thus, once a client is on board, it can be beneficial to get started with the exposure as soon as you can.

Programmed and Lifestyle Exposure: Encouraging Independence

Lifestyle exposures prepare the client for life after therapy

The illustrations of ERP in this chapter primarily illustrate *programmed* exposure in which the client implements planned exercises under your direction (e.g., at specific times and in particular locations). Yet it is also important for clients to engage in *lifestyle* exposure, which means making choices to take advantage of any opportunities to practice approaching (rather than avoiding) obsessional stimuli and choosing to be open to experiencing anxiety (rather than resisting it) –especially if these arise during valued activities. Encourage the client to be opportunistic and view spontaneously arising obsessional triggers as occasions to practice persisting with important activities while developing a healthier relationship with obsessions.

You can routinely remind clients that every choice they make regarding whether to approach or avoid an obsessional cue carries weight: Each time they choose to engage with such a situation without using rituals, they are strengthening new learning that will lead to long-term OCD symptom reduction. Yet, whenever a decision is made to avoid a potential lifestyle exposure situation, they are reinforcing their OCD-related fears.

As it becomes clear that the client has learned to correctly implement exposure independently, step back and encourage *becoming your own therapist*. This means allowing the client to design their own exposure tasks. This will prepare the client for life after therapy. Of course, the therapist still provides input regarding the nature of each exercise, and you will therefore continue to monitor the planning and implementation of these tasks.

Stylistic Considerations

Importance of Therapeutic Alliance

The quality of the relationship between therapist and client (including how well they align on therapeutic goals) is an important predictor of treatment outcome, and this holds true for ERP as well. Indeed, research consistently shows that a strong therapeutic alliance is an essential tool for promoting treatment adherence and successful outcomes in exposure therapy (Buchholz & Abramowitz, 2020). Accordingly, when conducting ERP, therapists should prioritize maintaining a strong connection and sense of collaboration with their clients throughout the process.

Remarks During Exposure Tasks

What to say (and what not to say) during exposure sessions

Offering appropriate observations, praise, encouragement, and support during exposure maintains the sort of rapport that is necessary for a successful outcome. Encourage the client to describe and talk about their thoughts and feelings. Also, foster conversation about what is being learned by doing exposures. If a client's anxiety happens to go down during the exposure, the following sorts of comments and open-ended questions can be helpful:

- "You're doing great facing this exposure head on. Remember, when you engage with a feared situation, you learn that you can manage it."
- "It looks like you're much less anxious now compared with when we started the session; and you haven't done any rituals. How do you explain that your anxiety is lower?"
- "This seems like it's getting easier for you. You're learning that obsessional thoughts and anxiety aren't as awful as you thought. Good for you!"
- "You were afraid that ______ would happen, but that hasn't happened. What do you make of that?"
- "You see, as we talked about before, you don't need to do rituals to get through this situation."

Even if the client's anxiety doesn't decrease during the exercise, convey understanding of how difficult exposure can be, and that with time and persistence, the exercises will become more manageable. Offer the following remarks:

- "Let's see if you can stick with the exposure even though it is difficult. You can do this! I know you can manage feeling the anxiety. You'll be glad you stuck with it."
- "Yes, the anxiety (fear, uncertainty, distress, disgust) is unpleasant and uncomfortable, but I know that you're strong - you can get through this. I have confidence in you!"
- "This time your anxiety did not decrease by much, but you still learned that anxiety does not have to go down for you to live your life. This is a very important lesson."

Avoid providing reassurance that exposure tasks are "not dangerous," that "nothing bad will happen," or that anxiety will definitely go down. These are not guarantees you can make, and more importantly, the client needs to discover this for themselves through their own experience (i.e., by doing the exposure). The example below illustrates helpful and unhelpful ways to address client requests for reassurance during exposure:

Client: Are you sure this is safe to do? Normal people wouldn't do a thing like this!

Unhelpful therapist response: Yes, it's OK. I promise. I wouldn't let anything bad happen to you. Just trust me.

Helpful therapist response: If you are asking me to guarantee you that the situation is absolutely safe, I can't do that. But I do know that all the evidence we have suggests that the risk is low enough that it's worth trying it out, even if it feels uncomfortable; and especially if doing this exercise will help with your OCD...

Dealing With Strong Urges to Ritualize

As clients begin response prevention, they may have difficulty with strong urges to ritualize. Reviewing how such urges are learned responses to obsessional cues, and how they are tolerable if resisted, is useful in helping the client refrain from rituals. The use of imagery can also be helpful, as in the example in Clinical Vignette 13 in which the client struggled with resisting compulsive urges to check door locks in her home.

Humor

The use of humor or laughter to lighten the mood during exposures may be appropriate and can be beneficial, although being playful is not always best in times of extreme distress. Follow the client's lead and ensure that remarks are relevant to the exposure situation and do not distract the client from the task. For instance, Clinical Vignette 13 is also an example of how some light humor on behalf of the therapist can help the client resist compulsive urges.

Clinical Vignette 13
Using Imagery to Manage Compulsive Urges

Therapist: Is there something you could imagine – it doesn't matter what the image is – that will grab you and help you resist? Perhaps you could imagine spraying the urge with a fire extinguisher or surfing on the urge until it crests and breaks.

Client: (smiling) I know what I can imagine – I could picture you standing in front of the door, waving your finger and shaking your head at me.

Therapist: That's great. Should I look mean?

Client: No, just having you there will help me stop checking.

Therapist: That sounds like a good plan.

Refining the Exposure List

Sometimes, important details of the client's obsessional fears do not become apparent until after the exposure list has been developed. Therefore, as treatment progresses, the therapist should remain alert for previously unidentified situations and stimuli that trigger obsessions or avoidance or that evoke compulsive rituals. Such situations should be incorporated into the exposure list.

Exposure Field Trips

The highly specific obsessions and avoidance behaviors of individuals with OCD often require that exposure exercises be conducted in public. Such field trips might include visiting funeral homes, cemeteries, restaurants, places of worship, hospitals, stores, the client's own home, driving, etc. If treatment is taking place in person (see Section 4.4.4), the therapist ideally has the flexibility to leave the office or meet the client at the site where such exposures can take place. If not, perhaps a well-coached support person can accompany the client on such trips. If treatment is occurring virtually, or in a hybrid fash ion, the session can take place with the client "on location" for the exposure (and the therapist joining virtually). If that is not feasible, another final option is for the client to check in with the therapist by phone during or following the exposure task.

Usually, exposures in public places can be conducted anonymously. The therapist and client should plan in advance how the exercise will proceed so that directives can be kept to a minimum in public. Conspicuous behaviors such as touching or rearranging items should be performed as discreetly as possible so as not to draw undue attention. Unforeseen difficulties, such as high levels of anxiety or a persistent sales clerk, can be managed by leaving the scene, regrouping, and returning another time. In some situations, it may be ideal to call ahead before visiting exposure situations. For example, one of the authors asked a client to call ahead to let a funeral home manager know that we would be dropping by. The client explained that the purpose of this visit was to help her overcome her fears of funerals. When a cover story and plans for various contingencies (e.g., running into a friend) are discussed ahead of time, we find that most clients are willing to go out in public to conduct exposure with their therapist.

4.1.8 Ending Treatment

This section discusses a number of issues that should be addressed toward the end of therapy.

Deciding on When to End Treatment

The following are often signs that it is appropriate to consider ending treatment in the near future:

- The client is able to completely (or almost completely) refrain from rituals.
- The client is able to design and implement exposures with minimal (or no) therapist input or guidance.
- The client's daily routine is not (or only minimally) adversely impacted by OCD symptoms.

Summarizing Treatment Progress

Using the *ERP Therapy Summary* form (Appendix 10), review with clients the progress they have made, including where things were when they began therapy (e.g., looking back at original treatment goals, symptom measure scores, and exposure list) compared with where they are now (i.e., current degree of OCD interference) and what lessons clients have learned that they want to remember (e.g., main take-home points of ERP, what techniques they found most helpful). Discuss plans and goals for the future, including what exposures clients still want to tackle and address any questions about how to incorporate ERP into the client's daily life.

Concluding Response Prevention

Help the client end response prevention and return to "typical" behavior

As the last session nears, begin to discuss appropriate checking, cleaning, arranging, or praying behaviors. As a rule, if such behaviors are performed in response to fears of negative consequences, they are probably rituals. Some examples of guidelines for resuming "typical" behavior after treatment appear below.

- Limit showering to one 10-minute shower per day. A second shower is permitted if there is extreme perspiration and body odor, or before getting dressed to go out (e.g., to a formal event). During any shower, wash each body part only once.
- Limit handwashing to 20 seconds triggered by activities such as using the restroom, eating, and when hands are visibly soiled (not simply because one "feels" contaminated).
- Once the door is closed, turn the handle once to make sure it is firmly locked. Otherwise, no returning to check is allowed.
- If a client genuinely does not know the answer to a question (e.g., how often people typically wash their bedding) they can ask a trusted support

person for input. However, if deep down they know the answer, they should refrain from asking for reassurance.

Assessing Treatment Outcome

Obtain posttreatment ratings of symptom severity to accurately document progress in treatment

In addition to informally assessing progress, evaluation of treatment outcome should include readministration of symptom measures (e.g., DOCS) and measures of general functioning (e.g., WSAS). Most clients will report some residual symptoms and impairment. Emphasize that some intrusions and repetitive behaviors are a part of everyday life for most people, so such experiences will likely never completely be absent. However, treatment has helped the client learn to respond to obsessional stimuli in new, healthy ways while continuing to engage in life's activities. Distress and functional impairment can be minimized with continued practice of the skills learned in treatment. In addition, there are self-help resources available for individuals with residual OCD symptoms following treatment (e.g., Abramowitz, 2025).

Continuing Care

Some clients desire additional treatment. As a general rule, those who have made little progress after 16 to 20 sessions of well-conducted ERP are unlikely to benefit further by adding additional sessions and might best consider taking a break from therapy and returning at a later date (additionally, see Section 4.5.13 about considering a higher level of care). Attending a support group run by a local affiliate of the International Obsessive-Compulsive Disorder Foundation (https://iocdf.org/ocd-finding-help/supportgroups/), if available, is another good option. If residual OCD symptoms are minimal, yet there is concern about possible relapse, follow-up sessions can be considered. Alternatively, a less formal strategy involving less frequent (perhaps monthly booster sessions) appointments could be undertaken. In such sessions, therapists can check in with clients about any important life updates, ask what skills clients have been practicing well and what progress they have made toward their long-term goals, identify where they are running into roadblocks, and problem solve ways to tackle them (e.g., brainstorming exposure exercises).

Preparing for Stressors

Clients should expect to experience residual OCD symptoms from time to time. Often, these are triggered by increased life stress, such as in the midst of occupational or family conflict, following a death or serious illness in the family, traveling, or around the time of childbirth. Help the client identify potential high-risk periods during which they should be ready to apply the techniques learned in therapy. Discuss warning signs for how the client can recognize things are not going well, and what skills clients can implement to get back on track.

4.2 Mechanisms of Action

A variety of different mechanisms have been proposed to explain how ERP works. There is no one agreed-upon mechanism, and rather it is likely that many of these processes of change are at play. These include (1) anxiety reduction (i.e., habituation) within and between sessions; (2) acceptance and willingness to experience obsessions, anxiety, and uncertainty; and (3) cognitive change – including (a) correcting mistaken beliefs about the need for rituals to keep one safe or to manage anxiety, as well as (b) fostering increases in self-efficacy.

First, from a learning theory perspective, ERP provides an opportunity for the extinction of conditioned fear responses. This approach views obsessional thoughts (and their triggers) as conditioned stimuli that provoke fear as a conditioned response. It conceptualizes avoidance, compulsive rituals, and other safety behaviors as strategies used to cope with or reduce obsessional fears, and these maladaptive coping strategies are negatively reinforced by the immediate (albeit temporary) reduction in distress they engender. Traditionally, the efficacy of ERP was understood in terms of *emotional processing theory* (EPT; Foa et al., 2006; Foa & Kozak, 1986), which credits initial fear activation followed by habituation (both within and between sessions) as the mechanisms of improvement. The basic assumptions of EPT, however, are not consistently supported by the research evidence (Craske et al., 2014). Specifically, successful habituation during exposure sometimes fails to predict long-term outcomes, and successful outcomes can occur in the absence of habituation.

Inhibitory learning is a proposed mechanism of fear extinction

Numerous developments in research on learning and memory relevant to exposure and extinction point to *inhibitory learning* as the mechanism of extinction (e.g., Craske et al., 2014). From the inhibitory learning perspective, the original threat-based association between the conditioned and unconditioned stimulus (e.g., "floors cause sickness" and "uncertainty about the future is intolerable") remain intact during exposure, while competing safety-based associations (e.g., "floors are generally safe" and "uncertainty is manageable") are formed. The goal of ERP for OCD, then, is to optimize the likelihood that the new safety-based associations will inhibit access to, and retrieval of, the older threat-based associations. In other words, the goal is to maximize the strength, durability, and generalization of the learning that takes place during exposure. The degree to which threat-based *versus* safety-based associations are expressed after finishing treatment depends on the strength of inhibitory learning across time and in different contexts. The descriptions and illustrations of ERP in this chapter incorporate numerous techniques and suggestions for maximizing inhibitory learning such as conducting exposures in a random order, combining multiple fear cues, consolidating what was learned following exposure, etc. (For more information please see Jacoby & Abramowitz, 2016).

Increasing acceptance of fear, uncertainty, and disgust also has clinical value in treating OCD and complements the goal of inhibitory learning (Jacoby & Abramowitz, 2016). To the degree that clients are willing to experience distress (e.g., "Anxiety and uncertainty are a part of life, so I'm better off learning to accept that I can't know for sure if every building I enter is 100% asbestos free"), inhibitory associations can be more robustly acquired ("I can push myself to go into older buildings and learn that I can manage this acceptable risk"). Increasing acceptance of fear, disgust, and uncertainty also reduces the likelihood that an inevitable unexpected encounter with one of these experiences in a new context (e.g., once treatment has ended) will lead to the return of fear and a relapse. This approach is consistent with the idea of willingness to experience obsessions, anxiety, uncertainty, and doubt from an ACT approach.

From a cognitive perspective, ERP corrects maladaptive beliefs that underlie OCD symptoms (e.g., overestimates of threat) by presenting the client with information that disconfirms these beliefs. Cognitive and educational interventions aim to modify such cognitions via a verbal-linguistic route, whereas ERP accomplishes the same goal experientially. Response prevention teaches clients that their anxiety is manageable even without time-consuming and costly rituals, and that their anxiety will not continue forever. ERP also facilitates self-efficacy by helping clients master their fears, learn to trust themselves, and continue to engage in everyday life without having to rely on avoidance or safety behaviors.

4.3 Efficacy and Prognosis

There is excellent scientific evidence of the efficacy of CBT for OCD

Numerous research trials evaluating the efficacy of exposure-based CBT for OCD consistently show that clients who complete this treatment achieve clinically significant and durable improvement. Average improvement rates are typically from 50% to 70% in these studies (Ferrando & Selai, 2021; Olatunji et al., 2013). A review of 24 trials (involving 1,134 study clients) indicated that CBT (primarily using ERP) was substantially more effective than comparison treatments (e.g., relaxation, anxiety management training, waiting list, medication) immediately following therapy (effect size = 0.75; Ferrando & Selai, 2021). Another meta-analysis of 16 studies found that CBT was moderately more effective at long-term follow-up (effect size = 0.43; Olatunji et al., 2013). These trials indicate that the effects of CBT are due to the specific cognitive and behavioral techniques (i.e., ERP) over and above any effects of nonspecific factors common to all interventions, such as the therapeutic relationship and spontaneous improvement. Moreover, the effects of CBT are not limited to highly selected research samples or to treatment delivered in specialty clinics. *Effectiveness studies* conducted with nonresearch clients (e.g., Franklin et al., 2000; Juel et al., 2025) have shown that around 80% of clients who complete CBT achieve clinically significant improvement. While CBT is effective for most people with OCD, about 20% do not respond and about 15–20% drop out of therapy (Ong et al. 2016). Factors associated with poor outcome (e.g., severe depression) are discussed in Section 3.4.

4.4 Variations and Combinations of Methods

4.4.1 Variants of ERP Treatment Procedures

There is a relationship between treatment outcome and how ERP is delivered along four parameters. First, better short- and long-term outcome is achieved when treatment involves in-session exposure practice that is supervised by a therapist, as compared with when all exposure is performed by the client as homework assignments. In fact, the number of hours of therapist-directed exposure is positively correlated with outcome. Second, combining situational and imaginal exposure is superior to situational exposure alone. Third, programs in which clients completely refrain from rituals during the treatment period produce superior immediate and long-term effects compared with those that involve only partial response prevention. Finally, compliance with instructions to homework exposure assignments between sessions is a predictor of positive outcome (Wheaton & Chen, 2021), which highlights the importance of exposure practice outside the session (i.e., the more work clients put into ERP, the more they get out of it).

In addition, it is essential that clients understand the rationale for using the various techniques discussed in this book. Research suggests that clients will be able to better apply and maximize benefit from ERP when they comprehend the conceptual basis for these strategies, perceive the treatment rationale to be credible, and expect to see improvement as a result.

4.4.2 Combining Medication and ERP

Research suggests that medication neither adds to, nor detracts from, the effectiveness of ERP for OCD

The concurrent use of ERP and SRI medication for OCD is common in clinical settings. The available research indicates that whereas adding ERP to SRIs tends to yield superior outcomes compared with SRIs alone, adding SRIs neither improves nor attenuates the efficacy of ERP (e.g., Foa et al., 2005). Thus, ERP is an excellent augmentation strategy for individuals with OCD who remain symptomatic despite adequate trials of SRI medications (but not necessarily the other way around). However, there may be certain clients who are unmedicated and who struggle with the ability to tolerate high levels of anxiety, who may benefit from a psychiatry consult to see whether an SRI could help dial down the intensity of the client's anxiety even slightly, such that they can more fully engage in ERP. If clients are prescribed fast-acting antianxiety medications (e.g., benzodiazepines), an important point of consideration is how clients are using these medications – if a client is taking an antianxiety medication at regular intervals (e.g., at bedtime to facilitate sleep), this may not interfere with ERP; however, if they are taking such medications on an "as needed" basis (e.g., when in the presence of obsessional triggers such as before or during exposure exercises), this can inadvertently contradict the goals of exposure therapy to be willing to experience fear and anxiety.

4.4.3 Involving Significant Others in Treatment

As has already been mentioned, for clients involved in close relationships (e.g., who are married), involving a significant other in ERP can have benefits; especially if the client is having difficulty completing exposure practices independently. The partner should attend treatment sessions and be introduced to the treatment approach and taught how to assist with exposure exercises by serving as a coach. This role includes offering emotional support to the client and providing gentle, but firm reminders not to ritualize. Train the partner to ensure that fears are adequately tested, and rituals resisted, during exposures. Emphasize helping the client get through the obsessional anxiety, as opposed to the partner trying to alleviate this distress.

There are four phases of partner-assisted exposure

In their couple-based CBT program for OCD, Abramowitz and colleagues (2013) divide the process of partner-assisted exposure into four phases and incorporate communication skills in each phase to help couples complete the exercises as a team. In session with the couple, you can introduce the four phases and then work through an exposure practice as follows:

Phase 1: Discussing the Exposure Task

Begin by helping the client and partner clarify the specifics of the exposure task. Both parties are encouraged to discuss how each is feeling about the upcoming practice (e.g., what is the client with OCD most worried about) and to identify potential obstacles. The client is helped to specify how they would like the partner to help with the exercise.

Phase 2: Approaching the Feared Situation

The second phase involves approaching and engaging with the exposure item. Encourage the client to express their feelings to the partner, who listens carefully and reflects these feelings instead of offering advice or solutions (e.g., "I can tell that you're feeling anxious about this exposure. I know this is challenging"). If the client becomes anxious, the partner acknowledges this, empathizes with the distress, and uses praise to reinforce the client's hard work (e.g., "You're doing great. I'm really proud of you!"). The partner continues to compliment the client on handling the situation throughout the exercise and avoids making negative statements. The partner also resists the temptation to distract the client, provide reassurance, or use any other anxiety reduction strategies.

Phase 3: Dealing With Intense Anxiety

If the client experiences intense distress during exposure, they are to communicate this to their partner. In turn, the partner acknowledges that exposure is challenging but that the client can get through it. If the client absolutely cannot continue with the exposure, a brief timeout can be taken during which the partner provides support in ways the client would like (but *not* using reassurance, rituals, or accommodation behaviors, if possible). The two parties also discuss what went wrong and how they can approach resuming the exposure. If the client with OCD decides to stop, ultimately it is their decision (e.g., partners may say, "I know that was hard, but you tried. We can try again another day").

Phase 4: Evaluation

Teach the parties to communicate with each other about how the exposure went. How did the client feel about the experience and the partner's coaching? What went well, and what could be improved next time? The partner should let the client know how they felt and, when appropriate, provide praise for a job well done (e.g., "I really love how hard you're working on this"). And the person with OCD should be sure to appreciate their partner for taking the time and energy to fight OCD alongside them.

For many partners, assisting with ERP and seeing a loved one experience anxiety is upsetting. In a manner of speaking, the partner is undergoing a form of ERP as well, allowing the client's distress to continue rather than reducing it by accommodation. Consequently, it is important to support the partner as well, both for being an effective coach and for tolerating the client's distress. Additional details regarding couple-based CBT for OCD can be found in Abramowitz et al. (2013).

4.4.4 In-Person Versus Virtual Treatment Delivery

In-person and virtual ERP have pros and cons. Various factors should guide the choice

Although virtual platforms have been used in the treatment of OCD for some time, the COVID-19 pandemic significantly accelerated their adoption and highlighted their potential to provide continuous, effective care when in-person sessions were not possible. Indeed, research suggests that virtual ERP can be just as effective as in-person therapy (e.g., Lisi et al., 2024). Accordingly, clinicians and clients have both options when it comes to modes of treatment delivery.

We recommend taking into account the following factors when deciding whether to use in-person, virtual, or a hybrid approach.

Severity and type of OCD symptoms: For clients with severe symptoms or those requiring hands-on interventions (e.g., being able to model an exposure for contamination concerns), in-person treatment will likely be more effective. Symptoms that necessitate exposures to specific environmental triggers (e.g., hospitals, children's playgrounds) may also be better suited for in-person sessions where both therapist and client can be present. Conversely, virtual therapy can be effective for more moderate cases or for symptoms that can easily be addressed through remote exposures (e.g., imaginal exposures). Additionally, virtual treatment can allow clients to practice exposure sessions in their own home (e.g., with their own bathroom, stove, etc.) with the therapist joining virtually, to facilitate generalization of learning to their real-world contexts.

Geographical and logistical considerations: Virtual treatment offers greater flexibility and convenience, enabling clients to access therapy from the comfort of their homes and at more flexible times. Clients living in remote areas, those with limited access to transportation, or those with mobility issues may find virtual therapy more feasible, as they eliminate travel time and offer greater scheduling flexibility.

Technological proficiency and access: Both client and therapist need reliable Internet access and familiarity with virtual platforms for teletherapy to be effective. Those lacking the necessary technology or comfort with digital tools or those who lack privacy at home might prefer in-person treatment.

Therapeutic relationship: Building a strong therapeutic alliance can be more challenging in a virtual setting. Therapists might find it challenging to fully assess and respond to nonverbal cues in virtual sessions, and clients who value face-to-face interaction and nonverbal communication might benefit more from in-person sessions. Others may find virtual interactions equally effective.

Personal preferences: Individual preferences play a significant role in the outcome of therapy – even skill-based interventions like ERP. Some clients may feel more comfortable and open in a virtual setting, while others may thrive in the structured environment of an in-person session.

A hybrid approach can offer the best of both worlds, allowing for flexibility and personalized care based on the client's evolving needs. For instance, initial intake sessions could either be conducted virtually (to minimize travel logistics) or in person (to foster a strong initial therapeutic alliance), followed by several in-person exposures to conduct exercises in a controlled environment and facilitate modeling exposures. Finally, treatment could progress with virtual exposures with clients in their real-world environment to up the ante and generalize learning.

4.5 Problems in Carrying Out the Treatment

Box 4 lists common problems that arise during ERP for OCD. Suggestions for managing such obstacles are provided below.

4.5.1 Negative Reactions to the Cognitive Behavioral Model

Some clients hold the belief that since OCD symptoms are caused by a genetic, neurobiological disturbance, or chemical imbalance, *talk therapy* won't be helpful. Because negative reactions to the cognitive behavioral model can lead to premature discontinuation, any doubts about the model should be discussed. Highlight the fact that the cognitive behavioral model was developed to explain the *maintenance* of OCD symptoms, not necessarily its causes (therefore, the ERP approach is not incompatible with a biological approach). You might also point out that studies show ERP has effects on brain functioning.

Box 4
Common Obstacles in ERP for OCD

- Negative reactions to the cognitive behavioral model
- Nonadherence
  - Noncompliance with exposure instructions
  - Noncompliance with response prevention instructions
  - Continued use of avoidance and subtle rituals
- Arguments between therapist and client
- Family accommodation
- Therapist's inclination to challenge the obsession
- Hijacking psychoeducational and cognitive therapy techniques to get reassurance
- Using exposure to control anxiety
- Intolerable anxiety levels during exposure
- Absence of anxiety during exposure
- Therapist discomfort with conducting exposure exercises
- Clients asking therapists for reassurance
- Reluctance to share intrusive thoughts
- Considering a higher level of care

4.5.2 Nonadherence

Improvement in ERP is directly related to client adherence to treatment instructions

The most common obstacle encountered in ERP for OCD occurs when a client is unwilling or unable to follow through with treatment instructions. Many adherence problems can be circumvented by ensuring that the client clearly understands the rationale for using these techniques. On occasion, this information needs to be reviewed with clients. You should also actively involve the client in the treatment planning process. There are a few ways in which nonadherence can occur which we review next.

Noncompliance With Exposure

If a client does not complete exposure tasks (e.g., homework assignments), inquire as to why this is. Sometimes the problem can be addressed with simple problem solving (e.g., time management). Also, make sure the exposure task itself is a good match to the client's obsessional fears and is a task that will improve their quality of life. If not, the client might perceive the exercise as irrelevant. If high levels of anxiety prompt refusal or "shortcuts" (e.g., subtle avoidance, rituals) during exposure, review the treatment rationale and emphasize that an important goal of treatment is anxiety acceptance. Cognitive strategies can also be used to identify and address maladaptive beliefs about anxiety that might underlie reluctance to engage with the feared stimulus (e.g., that anxiety will persist forever and spiral out of control).

Modifying the exposure list and adding items the client would be willing to try might be appropriate if the client may otherwise discontinue treatment.

Postpone exposures only as a last resort, because doing so can reinforce anticipatory anxiety and avoidance. Instead, start a discussion about the client's goals for treatment and how postponing exposures may conflict with values the client wishes to pursue (such as self-image, happiness, success, and being able to spend more time with friends and family). When a lack of progress in treatment is perceived as conflicting with important personal goals, it can increase motivation for change.

If, however, it becomes a pattern that a client is not completing homework exercises agreed upon at the previous session, a discussion may be needed about whether treatment should continue. In particular, in our experience it can be worse to continue ERP when actual ERP is not being done; in this situation, the client's lesson from treatment is that this approach does not work for them:

Therapist: It sounds like you may not be ready to tackle this exercise right now. You may remember that at the beginning of this treatment I referred to my role as being like a coach. And as your coach, I want to be honest with you that unless we make some changes, you're not going to see the benefits you want from treatment. As a reminder, the more you put into this treatment approach, the more you get out of it, and the last couple of weeks I know it has been challenging for you to attempt the exposure assignments at home. We could continue problem solving how to make that happen, but I also want to discuss with you whether this is truly the right time for you to be doing this kind of treatment. My concern is that if we continue down this path, your take-home message is going to be that ERP doesn't work for you. And I do really think this approach could help you! But right now, we're not really doing ERP. So, in these situations, it can be better to pause ERP and to resume another time down the road when you're ready to really take this on rather than to do it only partway. What do you think?

This discussion may lead to the client countering with why ERP is important to them in a way that results in recommitting to treatment. Or they may say that they have also been wondering if now is truly the right time for them to do ERP. In such a case, you can encourage them to take a break from treatment and come back when they are ready.

Noncompliance With Response Prevention

If the client is having difficulty refraining from compulsions, you can use motivational interviewing techniques to examine the pros and cons of engaging in rituals. For example, a client might identify that when they return home to check the stove, they feel a (temporary) reduction or relief in anxiety (pro). But cons they might verbalize include: (1) checking makes them less certain of themself, not more certain, (2) family members have become frustrated with repeated reassurance seeking, (3) being constantly preoccupied with needing to know everything takes up mental energy, etc. By the end of such a list, clients might find that the cons outweigh the pros, and they themselves are presenting compelling reasons for change.

If the client is deliberately concealing ritualistic behavior that was specifically targeted in the treatment plan, explain the implications of this problem for treatment outcome in the following way:

Therapist: Your wife emailed to tell me that you changed your clothes several times last weekend after going in the basement. She felt I needed to be aware of this because she was concerned that you weren't following the instructions we all agreed to at the beginning of therapy. In our joint session together, we all agreed that if problems come up, you were going to get help from your wife instead of doing rituals. Let's talk about this.

If the client makes a renewed agreement to adhere to the treatment instructions, the issue can be dropped. However, if repeated infractions occur, remind the client of the rationale for response prevention and raise the possibility that now is not the best time to undergo treatment. For example:

Therapist: It seems that right now you aren't able to stop your rituals as we had agreed at the beginning of treatment. Remember that each time you do a ritual you are preventing yourself from learning that you can handle the obsessional distress. If this is too difficult for you right now, perhaps this is not the right time for you to be doing this kind of treatment.

Continued Use of Avoidance and Subtle Rituals

Clients sometimes adopt covert tactics for avoiding or neutralizing obsessional distress even after stopping their overt rituals. These rituals can be so subtle that clients may not even be aware they have made such a substitution. Examples include the use of brief actions (e.g., quickly wiping hands instead of washing) or mental rituals (e.g., self-reassurance instead of asking others for reassurance). Although the client might not realize that these behaviors are interfering with treatment, they are functionally equivalent to overt compulsive rituals: They interfere with learning to manage obsessional situations and internal experiences (e.g., anxiety). Periodically inquire about such *mini rituals*, especially if highly anticipated exposures seem to be easy for the client. For example, "Now that you've stopped your compulsive rituals, are you doing any other subtle things to relieve anxiety?" Given that these rituals are at times unobservable, it is important that client and therapist work as a team to combat them.

4.5.3 Arguments

It is important to avoid arguing with clients about the treatment instructions

Some clients become argumentative about the "strictness" of response prevention rules or the "dangerousness" or "normality" of exposure tasks. You should resist the urge to get caught up in a debate with clients or to lecture them using logic (e.g., by appealing to probabilities); instead, use the Socratic method so that the belief-altering information is generated by the client themself.

In the example in Clinical Vignette 14, the client argues that speaking *one more time* with an infectious disease expert (Dr. B) would terminate his need for reassurance about the risk of catching HIV from public restrooms:

Clinical Vignette 14

Use of Socratic Dialog to Address Client Arguments

Client: I just have to ask Dr. B one more question about catching HIV from public toilets.

Therapist: I understand that you are anxious about this. Let's talk about that decision, though. You know that would be a compulsive ritual that we are trying to stop.

Client: But I need to know. I might have put myself at risk of catching HIV. You don't understand. I'm so worried.

Therapist: What has Dr. B told you in the past when you've asked her about these kinds of situations?

Client: That I'm not likely to catch HIV that way. But this time it's different. I *really* feel like I could have HIV. Please, just one more time. I have to ask her.

Therapist: Oh, so, each time you've asked Dr. B about HIV, she tells you that you probably have nothing to worry about. That's interesting. What do you think she'll say to you this time?

Client: She'll probably tell me the same thing.

Therapist: OK, so if you already know what she'll say, would you agree that the only reason for asking her again is just to hear ***her*** say it so that your anxiety and uncertainty is relieved?

Client: I guess so.

Therapist: Then wouldn't it be more helpful for you to use this opportunity to learn that you can tolerate this uncertainty and anxiety rather than always having to ask Dr. B. for reassurance whenever you think about HIV? After all, we've discussed how the reassurance seeking only makes OCD stronger because it only works temporarily.

Client: Yes. You're right. I see what you mean.

If discussions about the risks associated with exposure tasks become combative, summarize the discussion and agree with the client that their assertion *could* be correct (i.e., agree that some risk does exist); but that rather than analyzing the level of risk, it is better to practice managing uncertainty (e.g., using exposure). Do your best to refrain from debates over probability or the degree of risk. Such arguments reinforce the client's OCD patterns of spending too much time thinking about these issues, and they amount to little more than a playing out of the client's fruitless (ritualistic) attempts to gain reassurance. Such arguments can also rupture the therapeutic alliance. Moreover, when clients perceive that the therapist is frustrated, angry, or coercive, they often lose motivation (e.g., "You can't make me do this"). Instead, step back and recognize that the decision to engage in treatment is a difficult one, but ultimately let them choose whether or not to complete the exercise. This approach allows you to disengage from any sort of disagreements over whether an exercise is "safe" (and it is more likely to result in the client being willing to do the exercise vs. you having to convince them).

Clinical Pearl
When the Client Argues

When a client becomes argumentative (e.g., during exposure), it might indicate a rising level of distress. Instead of engaging in arguments about risk or "what is normal," the best strategy is to identify the problem and ask the client what they might suggest for resolving it. Have in mind how much it is useful to modify the therapy instructions without compromising treatment. Statements such as the following might also be helpful:

- You are here in treatment for yourself – not for me. So, I won't argue or debate with you. Doing the treatment is entirely your choice. You stand to get better by trying these exercises and learning how to handle the anxiety. But you are also the one who has to live with the OCD symptoms if you choose not to do the therapy or change it from what I'm suggesting. I'm here to help you get back to the life that you want.
- Remember that we both agreed on the treatment plan. I am here to help guide you, but to see improvements you will also need to put the work in too.
- I agree with you that there is *some* risk involved. The goal of treatment is to help you learn that you can be OK even in situations where it is impossible to have a complete guarantee of safety.
- I realize ***most*** people wouldn't go out of their way to do what I am asking you to do. But the therapy isn't about what people *usually* do. These tasks are designed to help you learn to manage acceptable levels of risk and uncertainty and to manage your OCD. Going above and beyond what people usually do is sometimes the most effective way to get over OCD (and I know you can do it!).
- Ultimately the decision is up to you, and I know this is a difficult one. Yet, if you are going to get over OCD, you have to confront uncertainty and find out that you can manage the risk.

4.5.4 Persistent Family Accommodation of OCD Symptoms

Accommodation can hinder treatment outcome

Accommodation of OCD symptoms by an intimate partner, other relative, or friend can hinder treatment outcome. If this is occurring, work with the client and accommodating individual together to help them change these interaction patterns. Describe accommodation and its deleterious effects, noting that such behavior is often well intended (as we discuss earlier in this book; see Section 1.2.4). Then, help the parties choose an activity which has become hampered by OCD symptoms, and facilitate a discussion about ways to handle this situation by promoting the idea of exposure and anxiety acceptance, rather than relying on avoidance and compulsive rituals. In other words, help the parties build ERP techniques into their relationship. For example, a husband might resume using various rooms in the house that had been off-limits. A wife might stop checking doors and windows prior to coming to bed. The goal of these interventions is to work toward a life in which loved ones engage with the situations and stimuli that the person with OCD has been avoiding to practice experiencing the anxiety.

When encouraging a loved one not to accommodate a client's OCD symptoms, it is important to understand what function the accommodation plays in the relationship and address these issues. For example, accommodation might have become a major way in which the husband shows care, concern, and love for his wife. Keep an eye out for situations in which removing accommodation changes the relationship such that the parties feel less close to each other, or the client does not feel as loved by their partner, family member, or friend. Discuss with the parties what new ways they want to show their love, care, and concern for each other, instead of through accommodation of OCD symptoms.

4.5.5 Therapist's Inclination to Challenge the Obsession

Therapists occasionally fall into the trap of challenging the logic of clients' obsessional thoughts (e.g., "the impulse to attack an elderly person") rather than challenging the client's faulty beliefs *about* the obsessions. Clinical Vignette 15 highlights the distinction between these two approaches (Examples 1 and 2).

Intuitively, the obsession itself seems like a good target for cognitive techniques because it is a cognitive event and may be irrational. Yet, most clients already recognize the irrationality of their obsessions. So, direct challenges will have only a transient therapeutic effect. It is also likely that support people in the client's life have already tried this rationalizing approach, and it has not worked. Moreover, such challenges could turn into reassurance-seeking strategies used to neutralize the obsession. In contrast, challenging the *appraisal* of the obsession can give the client new information that is different from reassurance.

Another option is to use ACT metaphors (e.g., Passengers-on-the-Bus metaphor, in Section 4.1.5) to help the client gain some distance from their thoughts and see them as *thoughts*, not *facts*. Example 3 in the vignette 15 illustrates this option.

Clinical Vignette 15
Challenging Obsessions

Example 1: Challenging the obsession

Therapist: Which intrusive thoughts have been problems for you this week?

Client: Every time I am around my grandfather, I get these terrible images of attacking him. He's a frail old man, and I love him very much. But I can't stop thinking about beating him.

Therapist: Let's look at the evidence. What do you think the likelihood is that you will beat your grandfather?

Client: Pretty low. I've never done it before, even though I've thought about it a lot.

Example 2: Challenging faulty appraisals and beliefs

Therapist: Which intrusive thoughts have been problems for you this week?

Client: Every time I am around my grandfather, I get these terrible images of attacking him. He's a frail old man, and I love him very much. But I can't stop thinking about beating him.

Therapist: When these kinds of thoughts come up, how do you interpret them? What do they mean to you?

Client: They mean that I am a terrible person deep down. I mean who the hell thinks of killing their own grandfather!? I need to be careful that I don't do anything awful, so I avoid him.

Therapist: Let's look more closely at your beliefs about these unwanted thoughts. Where is the evidence that because you have violent thoughts, you're really a violent person? What do we know about who has violent thoughts?

Client: Well, you taught me that occasionally everyone has thoughts like I do. So, maybe these thoughts aren't as dangerous as I'm thinking they are.

Therapist: And is it really possible to have a guarantee of safety?

Client: No, you're right. I suppose I'll never know for sure what these thoughts mean and if I'll one day act on them. I know I need to get better at tolerating that uncertainty.

Example 3: Using an ACT metaphor

Therapist: Which intrusive thoughts have been problems for you this week?

Client: Every time I am around my grandfather, I get these terrible images of attacking him. He's a frail old man, and I love him very much. But I can't stop thinking about beating him.

Therapist: Sounds like you've got some really loud passengers on the bus this week. What are they yelling at you now?

Client: They're saying that I am a terrible person deep down because I'm thinking about killing my own grandfather. And they're saying I need to be careful that I don't do anything awful, and that I need to I avoid him.

Therapist: It sounds like you've got some options. You can pull the bus over and argue with the passengers; you could just drive the bus where they want to go so that they'll quiet down for you; or you could keep driving the bus in the direction you want to go – toward spending quality time with family – and just let the passengers yell at you. What do you want to do?

Client: I guess I need to keep driving if I'm going to overcome this problem. Spending time with my family is really important to me.

4.5.6 Hijacking Psychoeducational and Cognitive Interventions

Watch out for OCD hijacking psychoeducational and cognitive interventions

Some clients convert discussions about mistaken beliefs into reassurance-seeking rituals. For example, one client ritualistically repeated (3 times perfectly) the phrase "obsessional thoughts are normal" to reduce anxiety associated with his unwanted sexual images before feeling "ready" to begin an exposure. Others become preoccupied with identifying the *perfect* rational belief that *best* reassures them that feared consequences are impossible. The best way to sidestep these problems is to amplify uncertainty and maintain the focus on accepting this feeling. For example, emphasize that even the most perfect rational belief is still a guess and not a guarantee.

As a general rule, if the client uses psychoeducational information in a stereotypic way, or requires increasing clarification (e.g., rereading psychoeducation material to feel less distressed), the material is probably being used as a ritual (and clients may benefit from targeting uncertainty instead). In contrast, healthy use of cognitive techniques and education involves lessons that clients truly believe and can internalize, results in long-term changes in behavior, and allows the client to developing a healthier relationship with obsessional stimuli that lead to acting appropriately during exposure.

4.5.7 Using Exposure to Control Anxiety

Dangers of emphasizing habituation as a goal of exposure

If clients see the point of exposure too narrowly as a means of reducing anxiety via habituation, it can lead to using exposure techniques as another anxiety control strategy (i.e., functionally equivalent to rituals) that, ironically, will interfere with treatment response. Signs of this include clients seeming relieved when exposure practices are over, saying that they "know anxiety will go down by the time the exposure is over," and describing their use of exposure (or its goal) as a way of lessening anxiety. Emphasizing habituation as a goal of exposure can increase the chances of clients inadvertently exploiting exposure in this way. To minimize the likelihood of this occurrence, emphasize that the aim of exposure is to practice leaning into anxiety, intrusive thoughts, and uncertainty, to learn that such emotions are tolerable – not to reduce them. In other words, the aim is to help the client become *better* at having anxiety, not to *reduce* it. Therefore, a "bring it on" attitude is appropriate, rather than the client's "white knuckling" stance. This highlights the importance of continually assessing for discrepancies in treatment goals.

Relatedly, we would not recommend relaxation training or controlled breathing techniques to be used in the context of ERP. While these techniques might be used in treatments for GAD, for example, an issue with incorporating them into exposure-based treatments for OCD is that clients may come to rely on them in the context of an exposure exercise. Conducting relaxation during an exposure may then serve to artificially force their anxiety levels down in a way that for clients with OCD can become a ritual or safety behavior itself, which is counter to the ultimate goal of helping the client tolerate anxiety and assume a bring-it-on attitude.

4.5.8 Intolerable Anxiety Levels During Exposure

It is important that the client sees high levels of anxiety (and obsessions and uncertainty) during exposure not as signs that treatment is failing, but as normal occurrences that are best used as opportunities to practice coping and enhancing distress tolerance (i.e., the bring-it-on attitude). If, however, the client becomes extremely anxious or emotional during an exposure, and says they want to stop, the exercise can be paused and the client's concerns discussed. You might focus this discussion on acceptance of anxiety or uncertainty, to identify exaggerated beliefs about experiencing these feelings without ritualizing (i.e., have clients put their feelings into words). Ultimately, clients are the ones in the driver's seat, so as a last resort an alternate exposure can be substituted, with the understanding that the client will come back to the original task at a later time. If the client is concerned that therapy is not working because anxiety does not subside, it suggests the need to review the aim of exposure as fostering anxiety acceptance. If the client is discouraged, point out that they took an important step simply by choosing to enter the feared situation in the first place.

4.5.9 Absence of Anxiety During Exposure

If the client reports little or no distress during exposure, it could mean one of three things. First, the situation might no longer evoke anxiety. That is, the client's obsessional fear has been extinguished. This is most likely to occur toward the end of treatment. In such cases, you might skip to another exposure item or conduct exposure in a different context. A second explanation is that you have not incorporated the main anxiety-evoking aspect(s) of the feared situation into the exposure task. To troubleshoot, ask the client why the exercise does not evoke fear, or how it could be made more anxiety evoking. A third possibility is that the client has nullified the exposure with cognitive avoidance or rituals. For example, before conducting a driving exposure, one client called her neighbors to warn them to closely watch their children during the time she would be driving through the neighborhood streets. This absolved her of the responsibility for harm, and therefore she did not become anxious during the driving exposure. The use of such strategies indicates a problem in understanding the treatment rationale, or difficulties adhering to its principles, and must be addressed for clients to maximally benefit from therapy.

4.5.10 Therapist Discomfort With Conducting Exposure Exercises

Look out for your own negative beliefs and distress about exposures

Despite the well-known effects of ERP, many therapists – even those who have been trained in the delivery of exposure – either refrain from using this technique or use it suboptimally, so as to not subject clients to high levels of anxiety. Such therapists may hold negative beliefs about exposure, including that it is harmful, will disrupt the therapeutic relationship, is overly rigid, will lead clients to drop out of treatment, etc. Minimizing the intensity of exposure is associated with concerns about the adverse consequences of purposely confronting stimuli that will evoke high levels of discomfort (Deacon & Farrell, 2013). Recall, however, that the beneficial effects of ERP are well-documented (see Section 4.3 for more details). Reducing OCD in the long-run requires evocation of anxiety to learn how to manage this and other OCD-related inner experiences better. Also, exposure helps clients learn that their feared situations and thoughts pose acceptable levels of risk. Response prevention helps the client learn that time-consuming and embarrassing rituals are not necessary to prevent feared outcomes. In fact, when the rationale for ERP is clear and the treatment plan is set up collaboratively, doing this treatment prompts a supportive and highly rewarding working relationship which helps the client make considerable and long-lasting progress. Accordingly, therapists may need to build their own distress tolerance when conducting exposure by practicing sitting with clients' anxiety during in-session exposures and empathizing with their distress without trying to fix it. Such an approach can also facilitate therapist cognitive change regarding some of these negative beliefs of exposure.

4.5.11 Clients Asking Therapists for Reassurance

The challenge of clients with OCD asking therapists for reassurance was raised in section 4.1.6. However, sometimes a therapist's initial encouragement to stick with uncertainty may meet additional resistance from clients who are pressing for more information. Here therapists might choose to balance pushing back against OCD on the one hand, with maintaining the therapeutic alliance on the other. Specifically, therapists might choose to answer such questions only part way.

Example 1: "It is unlikely you will get sick from touching this doorknob, but I can't give you a 100% guarantee."

Example 2: "From everything you've told me, it sounds as though you're the type of person who cares a lot about other people, and does whatever you can to not harm others. Knowing 100% for sure whether you might have accidentally harmed someone in the past is never really possible, and so one thing we can work on is starting to trust yourself a bit more."

4.5.12 Reluctance to Share Intrusive Thoughts

Checklists of obsessions can normalize unacceptable thoughts and facilitate client disclosure

Bear in mind that you might be the first person that your client has shared their intrusive thoughts with, and opening up can be challenging for some clients. Alternatively, many clients have had negative experiences with previous providers, in which they may have shared such thoughts, and the therapist inadvertently fueled their OCD by misinterpreting these thoughts as facts (e.g., a clinician thinking that an ego-dystonic violent thought is a sign that a client is dangerous), so some reluctance can also be understandable. Clients will be more willing to open up, the more comfortable and willing therapists appear to hear what they have to share. Specifically, you can assure your client that OCD is one of your specialties and that you have heard all kinds of different bothersome thoughts from clients before (and convey the message that you will be able to hear about these thoughts without any shock or judgment).

Second, as previously mentioned in Section 1.7.3, when introducing the Y-BOCS checklist you can make clear to clients that this is a list of very common obsessions and compulsions. While clients may be more reluctant to spontaneously disclose obsessions about some of these taboo topics, they are much more likely to endorse them when they are already on your checklist.

If the client is still reluctant to share, treatment could begin with other obsessions and compulsions before circling back around to the avoided topic in order for the client to gain some trust in you. Some exposures can even be done to these thoughts before the client is willing to share them with you (e.g., you could have them write the thoughts down on paper as an exposure even if they are not willing to show you the paper). However, it is also important to convey how helpful for treatment it is for clients to be able to share this information, since shame tends to remain or worsen if these thoughts are unspoken. Furthermore, clients who are unwilling to share these thoughts may do so out of fear that you will determine the thoughts are not really OCD (e.g., that they are indeed a dangerous or violent person), and such beliefs cannot be challenged if you do not know the content of the client's thoughts.

4.5.13 Considering a Higher Level of Care

There are a few indicators that you might consider a higher level of care for a client. First, if you have been following the guidelines in this book and the client has not improved in 8–12 sessions (i.e., you are monitoring their scores on measures like the DOCS, and the scores have not reduced), referrals to a higher level of care may be needed. Additionally, if the OCD is so impairing that (a) the symptoms are interfering with the client being able to attend weekly sessions (e.g., they are canceling due to avoidance or showing up 45 minutes late because they cannot stop performing rituals) or complete homework assignments without therapist support, and/or (b) their functioning is impaired to the point at which they are at risk of failing a semester of courses, losing their job, or having their spouse leave them, for example (or if this has already happened), these might be signs that taking a medical leave to pursue more intensive treatment would be warranted.

4.6 Multicultural Issues

4.6.1 International Presentations of OCD

Research supports the generalizability of the CBT model cross-culturally

OCD is observed in individuals worldwide, and culture often plays a role in shaping the presentation of obsessions and compulsions, which has bearing on treatment. In a series of studies, a large group of investigators collected data from 777 participants in 13 countries on 6 continents (Clark & Radomsky,

2014; Radomsky et al., 2014). Although the majority of participants in each country experienced obsession-like intrusions, those in the United States reported the highest frequency, and those in Argentina, the lowest. There were differences in the *content* of intrusions: participants from Sierra Leone reported the highest frequency of contamination-related intrusions, while those from the United States and Turkey reported the highest number of religious intrusions. Cross-culturally, doubt was the most common type of intrusion. Thus, while the experience of unwanted intrusions is universal, there are differences in the content of such thoughts across cultures.

As predicted by the cognitive-behavioral model of OCD, the relationship between appraisals and thought frequency were comparable across countries; and the more an intrusion was appraised as highly unacceptable, significant, and threatening, the more it was also rated as distressing and uncontrollable (Clark & Radomsky, 2014; Radomsky et al., 2014). Moreover, the tendency to use reassurance seeking or another compulsive ritual to control an intrusion predicted greater frequency of distressing intrusions cross-culturally. Avoidance, distraction, thought replacement, and thought stopping, however, were relatively unrelated to the frequency or distress of intrusive thoughts. These findings support the generalizability of the cognitive behavioral model of obsessions cross-culturally and suggest that ERP should be the first-line psychological treatment worldwide (Clark & Radomsky, 2014; Radomsky et al., 2014).

Clinical observations and empirical studies indicate that obsessional content stems from matters which are culturally relevant to the individual, resulting in diverse symptom expression. In Europe, the United States, Australia, and Canada, contamination/cleaning, symmetry/ordering, taboo thoughts/mental compulsions, and doubt/checking are commonplace among those with OCD (e.g., Hunt, 2020). In Hispanic and Latin American people with OCD, contamination and aggression are among the most common obsessions. Among Indian samples, obsessions often concern contamination and pathological doubt, with greater gender differences in symptom dimensions. In East Asian samples, concerns about contamination and symmetry are prominent, with cultural differences between Japan and China: greater need for symmetry in China, and elevated concerns with contamination and aggression in Japan (e.g., Hassan et al., 2024). Less research is available from African cultures (Wilson & Thayer, 2020).

The presence of religious compulsions among individuals of different religions indicates that faith also influences OCD symptoms. Among Protestant Christians, contamination and taboo (e.g., blasphemous) obsessions predominate, along with washing and mental rituals. Among Catholics, an emphasis on perfectionism has been observed; and among Jews, themes of morality and divine retribution seem to appear in obsessions. Obsessions among Islamic individuals tend to focus on purity and religious themes (e.g., Inozu et al., 2017). OCD in Near Eastern countries tends also to reflect religious beliefs, as well as familial and societal values.

Clinical observations suggest that religious OCD symptoms may respond less well to ERP than do other presentations of the problem. Specifically, it might be difficult for a client or a clinician to distinguish between acceptable religious or moral behavior (and thoughts) versus OCD symptoms. Thus, cultural competence on the part of the therapist and a good understanding of a client's belief system are important (Abramowitz & Jacoby, 2014; Williams et al., 2020).

4.6.2 Justice-Based Treatment of OCD

Exposures should not contribute to minority stress

Clients with OCD commonly experience intrusive thoughts in which they doubt their sexual orientation or gender identity (e.g., "What if my relationship with my husband is a lie, and I'm supposed to be with women"), or in which they experience unwanted racist, homophobic, or transphobic intrusive thoughts (e.g., the urge to yell a racial slur in the middle of a meeting). These topics require special consideration to ensure that any exposures designed do not cause undue harm to the minoritized individuals who are identified in these obsessions. Specifically, ERP clinicians should eliminate exposures that contribute to minority stress and replace them with psychoeducation about minoritized identities, and exposures to neutral and positive stimuli and uncertainty, while still targeting core fears.

For example, if a client were afraid of losing control and saying a racial slur when interacting with individuals of other races, rather than reading, writing, and saying that word over and over again – which would serve to normalize the harmful slur and contribute to the minority stress of individuals from that racial group, including clinicians who may be working with the client – the client could instead practice talking to coworkers of other races at their office whom them have been avoiding and tolerating anxiety or uncertainty that the unwanted word would somehow slip out. As another example, rather than finding and talking to people who "look" transgender (or bringing a transgender colleague into an exposure as a confederate) – which would serve to tokenize such individuals (not to mention perpetuate the inaccurate belief that one's gender identity is the same as one's gender expression) – the client could instead attend a rally for members of the LGBTQ+ community and their allies and tolerate not knowing for sure the gender identities of those around them. Lastly, rather than writing an imaginal exposure involving the client having a sexual encounter with someone of the same sex and including details about feeling "disgusted" – which reinforces the belief that same-sex relationships are somehow gross or undesirable – the client could write an imaginal exposure about coming out and the consequence of doing so (e.g., loss of current romantic relationship, being labeled a "liar"). Each of these examples allows clients to engage with obsessional stimuli and practice tolerating anxiety and uncertainty, *without* harming individuals of minoritized groups in the process. For more reading on the topic of the justice-based treatment of OCD, see Pinciotti et al. (2022) and Williams et al. (2020).

5

Case Vignettes

This chapter presents examples of exposure lists and treatment plans (session-by-session descriptions of situational and imaginal exposure tasks) for different presentations of OCD. ERP in each of these four cases resulted in marked improvement in quality of life as a result of successful fear extinction and reduction in compulsive rituals. You can use these vignettes as templates for building treatment programs for your clients.

Case 1: Contamination Symptoms

Priya, a 36-year-old restaurant manager, feared contracting hepatitis. She avoided public transportation and touching surfaces like elevator buttons and handrails. Priya also avoided contact with other people and their personal items (cell phones, cutlery, etc.). Food and drink prepared by others also triggered obsessive fear. Priya washed her hands over 50 times each day and frequently changed her clothes to reduce her fears of contamination. If she could not avoid a perceived contaminant or had to delay washing or cleaning, Priya would try to suppress any thoughts of hepatitis germs and contamination, mentally reassuring herself that she was going to be okay. She also would mentally keep track of which objects in her home were considered "clean" versus "dirty." Even though Priya acknowledged that the likelihood of contracting hepatitis from everyday objects was very small, she stated that she would "rather be safe than sorry" and found the anxiety she experienced in the face of contamination-related uncertainty to be overwhelming and "too strong to manage."

Treatment began with a few sessions of information gathering, assessment, and treatment planning. Priya was on board with treatment and, although anxious about trying ERP, believed it was important to challenge herself to approach her fears. Her exposure list is shown in Table 8 (listed in ascending order of SUDs):

Table 8
Priya's Exposure List (With SUDS)

Item	SUDS
Elevator buttons	45
Using public transportation and touching handrails	55
Shaking hands with others	65
Other commonly touched surfaces (e.g., grocery carts, door handles)	70
Using public restrooms	70
Eating food prepared by someone else	75
Sharing cell phone with someone else	80
Sitting on public benches without cleaning them first	80
Handling money	85
Using shared office equipment	90
Using vending machines	95

Note. SUDS = subjective units of distress.

Priya's response prevention plan was as follows:

- Try to avoid contact with water, except for one 10-minute shower and one 2-minute tooth brushing each day. If washing cannot be avoided, she was instructed to re-approach stimuli from the exposure list.
- No cleaning items or objects.
- No mental reviewing or reassurance. "If I catch myself trying to review or reassure myself, I will focus on uncertainty about germs."

During the first exposure session, Priya practiced touching elevator buttons around the therapist's clinic building. She also shook hands with others in the building, such as support staff, security guards, and other professionals. She was encouraged to think about the possibility that she could contract hepatitis from these activities. Before beginning the exposure, Priya said that she thought she could only "stand" being in contact with these contaminants (and tolerating the associated contamination-related thoughts and uncertainty) for 5 minutes. Thus, she was very surprised that she was able to manage the distress these tasks provoked for more than 30 minutes. While conducting the exposure, Priya and her therapist also discussed distressing images of receiving a diagnosis of hepatitis, uncertainty about where people might have put their hands, and who might have touched the buttons she pressed (imaginal exposure). Between sessions, Priya practiced shaking hands and touching more elevator buttons, especially before eating, in a variety of different locations with varying level of difficulty (i.e., perceived dirtiness).

At the second exposure session, Priya and the therapist met at a bus stop and boarded a public bus. They rode the bus for 30 minutes and Priya touched the seat and handrails, maintaining contact with each for a period of several minutes. Back in the therapist's office, Priya created a recording of her description of "hepatitis germs" crawling all over her body and listened to the recording (imaginal exposure) without washing her hands. The aim in this session was to purposely provoke feelings of anxiety and uncertainty in order for Priya to learn that she could function even when she was feeling "dirty." Priya agreed that between sessions, she would ride the bus a few times, and also begin touching other commonly touched surfaces, such as grocery carts and doorknobs in a variety of places she had been avoiding, such as at work and in certain stores. She also practiced imaginal exposure using the recorded material. Priya was also encouraged to contaminate additional personal items at home with "germs" from the bus.

Public bathrooms were the focus of exposure session 3. Priya touched bathroom door handles, sink faucets, and soap dispensers, and maintained contact with these items for several minutes. She addressed her fear of toilets by sitting on the floor next to the bowl and touching the flusher and seat. For practice between sessions, she was instructed to sit on public toilets in various places she had been avoiding (e.g., work bathrooms) and allow herself to "bring on" the feelings of doubt about whether these restrooms were properly cleaned or had hepatitis germs. Imaginal exposure included images of such germs, as well as thoughts of uncertainty and severity of becoming ill.

For the fourth exposure session, Priya arranged to bring cookies and brownies that had been prepared by one of her neighbors whom she had been avoiding. Priya ate some of the food in the session and planned to practice eating more on her own during the upcoming week. Imaginal exposure to images of hepatitis was continued, and Priya practiced eating with her hands immediately after touching items that she had approached for exposure earlier in treatment (e.g., grocery carts). She repeated these and similar exercises each day between the fourth and fifth sessions.

The fifth session of exposure involved sharing her phone with the therapist by allowing the therapist to touch and speak into her phone. She placed her phone on various surfaces (floors, public chairs, railings) that she had been avoiding, and she refrained from washing her phone afterwards. Imaginal exposure to images of hepatitis germs was continued. By this point, Priya felt she was becoming less and less concerned about illness since none of the previous exposures had led to any problems. Priya described feeling genuinely (and pleasantly) surprised by this development.

At exposure session six, Priya reported that her urges to wash her hands and clean surfaces had significantly decreased during the previous week. She and the therapist met at a mall and practiced sitting on public benches, handling money, and generally touching more public surfaces that Priya had been avoiding or washing after contact. She was surprised at her ability to perform these activities with little distress, even with occasional thoughts of contamination and uncertainty about hepatitis. Priya decided that during the coming week, she would practice using shared office supplies and equipment at her restaurant, which she had still been avoiding.

At the seventh exposure session, Priya reported that she had had success using shared equipment at her restaurant and was feeling more confident in other areas of her life, such as running errands and using the bathroom if she was out. During the session, she and her therapist visited the vending machines on different floors of the clinic's office building, and Priya was able to touch these machines and eat food without washing.

Sessions 8 through 16 included repeated exposures to public bathrooms, handling money, and touching frequently touched public surfaces without washing, and then eating. Imaginal exposure to distressing thoughts and periodic contact with lesser contaminants was continued. Priya was also encouraged to continue "contaminating" additional personal items at home.

Case 2: Existential Obsessions

Armando, a 33-year-old real estate agent, experienced persistent unwanted obsessional thoughts and doubts of an existential nature, such as "What if I am not fulfilling my life's purpose?" "What if I have free will and I'm not making the right choices?" and "How do I know who I am supposed to be?" He reported that these ideas and questions were ever-present in his mind, and that they were especially activated when he had to make seemingly consequential decisions, such as at work or in his relationships. In response to these obsessions, he engaged in compulsive reading about philosophy on the Internet trying to get acceptable answers to these questions, or at least to help him better "understand" what they meant. He also did a lot of reassurance seeking with his wife and with his parents, whom he was close to. Armando reported having bouts of these types of OCD symptoms daily since he was a teenager, and that it was interfering with his marriage, although he was able to function well enough at work.

Armando's exposure list is shown in Table 9:

Table 9
Armando's Exposure List (With SUDS)

Item	SUDS
Consider recent decisions without researching or seeking reassurance	45
Discuss an existential question (with his wife) without trying to solve it	50
Think about not being able to know life's true purpose	60
Think about not fulfilling my life's true purpose	65
Make a decision (e.g., at work) without existential considerations	70
Read material about free will versus determinism without further research	75
Create a video about my existential doubts and watch without reassurance or research	80

Note. SUDS = subjective units of distress.

Armando's response prevention plan was as follows:

- No doing research about existentialism, free will and determinism, the meaning of life, or the like.
- No seeking reassurance by asking other people about existentialism, free will, the meaning of life, etc.

When Armando began treatment, he was in danger of losing his job because his attendance at work and his sales numbers were in decline due to OCD. Thus, he stated that he was determined to work hard in therapy.

At the first session, Armando's therapist introduced the ACT concept of *experiential avoidance* and helped Armando to consider that his OCD had three parts: (1) his unwanted intrusive thoughts, (2) his responses to the intrusive thoughts, and (3) the functional interference. Armando was able to understand that his existential obsessions arose from *normal* existential thoughts that most people experience, but that his persistent (yet futile) efforts to *fix* or *push away* these thoughts (i.e., compulsive rituals) were leading to obsessional preoccupation. Moreover, his rituals caused the reduction in his quality of life. The therapist, therefore, explained that the goal of therapy would be for Armando to learn a healthier relationship with his intrusive thoughts, rather than to make them disappear or to "resolve them." Armando was on board with this approach. Various ACT metaphors were used to illustrate the futility of trying to dismiss or resolve existential questions, and how *making room* for these thoughts while pursuing valued activities would help Armando function better in his various life roles.

Accordingly, ERP was conducted from within an ACT framework and the focus was less on SUDS and more on Armando's learning to be *open* to and *accepting* the ubiquity of existential thoughts. Exposure began with Armando addressing his obsession with making the "right" decisions based on his "life's purpose." Armando was asked to think about recent decisions he had made, without researching online or seeking reassurance from others. He reflected on choosing a new marketing strategy for a property listing, focusing on the discomfort of not verifying his choice through additional sources. Armando could not be certain that he had acted completely in line with his "purpose in life," yet instead of trying to figure this out, he practiced *making space* for this doubt while he went about his daily routine. Armando practiced similar exposures during the week between sessions with the therapist.

In exposure session two, Armando's wife was present, and Armando discussed an existential question with her without trying to find a solution. Specifically, he shared his recurring thought, "What if I am not fulfilling my life's purpose?" with her, focusing on the anxiety it provoked without asking for her reassurance or insights. Typically, Armando's wife would respond to such conversations either by trying to reassure Armando with logic or by becoming frustrated with Armando. The therapist helped the couple discuss the obsession in a healthier way that involved Armando's wife letting Armando know that she understood his anxiety and knew he was strong and could get through his distress independently. They also discussed how to use ACT metaphors, such as the Unwelcome Guest at the Party and the

Chessboard Metaphor to help Armando get through his distress, rather than ritualize.

During the third and fourth exposure sessions, Armando was helped to address his uncertainty about life's true purpose. The therapist guided him through a series of reflections on the impossibility of fully knowing his purpose, emphasizing the need to make room for the discomfort and doubt that this thought caused without turning to research or reassurance-seeking behaviors. Armando was also helped to think deeply about his fear of not fulfilling his life's true purpose (especially since it was impossible to know the true purpose in the first place). He reflected on past decisions and life paths he had not taken, practicing increasing his openness and willingness to experience the uncertainty these thoughts brought up without attempting to alleviate it through compulsive rituals.

The focus of the fifth exposure was making a significant work-related decision without considering existential implications. Armando decided on a new real estate investment strategy, deliberately avoiding thoughts about whether this choice aligned with his ultimate purpose and tolerating the resulting anxiety without seeking additional information or reassurance. At this point, Armando fully embraced the agenda of "letting go of the rope" instead of playing tug of war with his obsessional thoughts. He reported feeling more and more confident about making decisions even if he could not resolve his obsessional doubts.

For the sixth exposure, Armando read a challenging article on the issue of free will versus determinism, a topic that typically triggered his existential doubts. He engaged with the material without allowing himself to look up further explanations or ask others for their interpretations, practicing tolerating the uncertainty and anxiety that arose.

During the seventh exposure session, the therapist guided Armando to create a video where he spoke about his existential doubts. After recording the video, he watched it repeatedly, focusing on hearing his fears and uncertainties aloud without seeking reassurance or conducting further research. This exercise further aimed to increase his acceptance of his obsessive thoughts. Armando's wife also attended this session and reported that she and Armando had had virtually no reassurance-seeking conversations in the past few weeks and that their relationship had been improving.

Armando attended five more sessions with the therapist before deciding that he was doing well enough to discontinue treatment. These last exposure sessions involved further practice reflecting on recent decisions without seeking reassurance (e.g., he focused on his choice of a vacation destination for his family, resisting the urge to verify if it was the best choice or ask his family for their opinions multiple times), and focusing on the impossibility of fully knowing life's true purpose. During the final session, Armando reflected on his overall journey through therapy, acknowledging the persistent uncertainty and anxiety and reinforcing his ability to live with unanswered questions without engaging in compulsive behaviors.

Case 3: Relationship OCD

Stephanie, a 28-year-old woman who lived with her fiancé, Andrew, experienced debilitating doubts about her romantic relationship. These intrusions would often pop up when the two of them were spending quality time together (e.g., watching a TV show or having dinner with friends). Specifically, Stephanie would find herself starting to wonder: "Do I love Andrew?" "Is he the right person for me?" While she was fairly certain that she wanted to marry Andrew (and thus said yes when he proposed), she still struggled with lingering doubts about what if she'd made a mistake and if she was really ready to spend the rest of her life with him. Stephanie also engaged in time-consuming rituals such as testing herself to see if she was still as attracted to Andrew as she once was, by scrolling back in her phone to look at old photos from their first dates and mentally reviewing the details to see if doing so sparked the same emotions that the original moments once did. Many of Stephanie's other friends were getting married and committing to their long-term partners, and she wondered what was wrong with her that in comparison they all seemed so sure. Andrew was unaware that Stephanie was experiencing these obsessional thoughts. He had noticed recently that she had been avoiding being sexually intimate, but he attributed that to the stress of the wedding planning. And as the wedding approached, Stephanie presented to treatment because the doubts about how to move forward were escalating to the point that they were interfering at work and with her sleep. She lived in a rural part of her state, and so finding an ERP therapist within a 1-hr radius of her home was not possible. Thus, Stephanie conducted the following course of ERP solely over a secure telehealth platform.

Table 10
Stephanie's Exposure List (With SUDS)

Item	SUDS
Watch movie clips of happy couples without comparing my relationship with that in the story	40
Look at photos of us without testing myself to see if I feel the same	55
Being sexually intimate with Andrew without overanalyzing whether I am enjoying it	67
Watching movie scenes or listening to songs about breakups	75
Make final decisions in wedding preparations (e.g., commit to the caterer)	75
Write an imaginal exposure script in which I stay with Andrew and never know for sure if he's the right person	80
Write an imaginal exposure script in which I leave Andrew and never know for sure if I made a mistake	85

Note. SUDS = subjective units of distress.

Stephanie's exposure list included the following items (listed in Table 10 in ascending order of SUDS). At each session, the specific exposures to be conducted were determined collaboratively, based on interference with Stephanie's quality of life. Specifically, she expressed a strong desire to be able to improve her relationship with Andrew and to get back on track in planning their wedding. Thus, the order of exposure tasks to be completed was determined based on helping her reach these goals as quickly as possible.

Stephanie's response prevention plan was as follows:

- No overanalyzing the relationship
- No testing herself to see if she is still attracted to Andrew
- No mentally reviewing the pros/cons of their relationship
- No reassurance seeking from friends about their relationships or what they think of Andrew

At exposure session one, Stephanie practiced making a final decision in her wedding planning (i.e., choosing the bakery for her wedding cake). This exposure was important for her to tackle as soon as possible (even though it was a more anxiety-provoking task) because not making some of these decisions was beginning to cause problems (e.g., she was overdue on paying some wedding invoices, and she had lost out on opportunities such as her first-choice band because she could not reach a decision). Stephanie and Andrew had been to five different bakeries doing cake tastings, and Stephanie was afraid to commit to one as this brought her one step closer to marrying Andrew. She also found that the more cakes she tried, the more uncertain she was of which vendor to choose (and felt paralyzed by wanting to pick the *perfect* cake). Therapy focused on limiting her options and tolerating that the number of bakeries she had tried was "good enough" (i.e., not looking at additional bakeries), eliminating further procrastination by making a final decision in the session, and reducing reassurance seeking from others (i.e., refraining from asking her mom or Andrew one more time for their opinion, as they had already told her they were happy with the options, and it was her choice). Once she called and made the initial deposit on the wedding cake, Stephanie discussed with her therapist the idea of trusting her own opinions and decisions going forward. Between sessions, Stephanie worked on making several additional wedding-related decisions and crossing other items off her to-do list (e.g., paying an overdue deposit to the caterer).

The second session involved engaging with a variety of stimuli that Stephanie had been avoiding, including watching movie clips of happy couples (by using the screen share function on the telehealth platform), as well as listening to songs about breakups (she would typically change the channel if a breakup song came on). The exposures were arranged to help Stephanie demonstrate to herself that she could stick with the associated distress longer than she thought. She also practiced noticing if her mind began to overanalyze any similarities between the movie or song and her own relationship. She learned that such experiences, although uncomfortable, were manageable. Between sessions, Stephanie chose to watch a romantic comedy that Andrew had asked her to watch and to which she had previously said no because she was "too tired." She also refrained from changing the radio when songs about breakups and love inevitably came on.

Exposure session three involved Stephanie looking at a photo of her and Andrew from when they first started dating, without testing herself to see if she felt the same. She practiced talking about the memory in the photo with her therapist, as well as detailing the positive and negative aspects about the evening (without weighing the pros/cons, but simply allowing both to be there). The second half of the session was also reserved for planning a between-session exposure practice in which Stephanie wanted to resume sexual activity with Andrew. She and her therapist discussed the goal of being in the present moment without trying to test if she was still attracted to Andrew. They discussed how the overanalyzing itself would likely interfere with Stephanie's enjoyment of being intimate with her fiancé, and how by minimizing this ritual she could move in the direction of her values.

At the fourth and fifth sessions, Stephanie wrote imaginal exposure scripts both about the feared scenario that she would marry Andrew and never know for sure if he was the right person, as well as the scenario that she would leave him and never know for sure if she made a mistake. The goal was to "bring on" as much uncertainty as she could, sit with those doubts, and not try to resolve them. Stephanie made recordings of each script on her smartphone and listened to them in between sessions. Stephanie and her therapist discussed that the purpose of these exposures was not to prove or disprove whether Andrew was the "right person," since whether or not there was someone else out there who was better suited for her was unknowable.

The remaining sessions involved repeated exposure to the various items practiced previously, but in different contexts. By the end of treatment, Stephanie was able to return to activities that she used to do that she had been avoiding (e.g., being sexually intimate with Andrew), made measurable progress on her wedding planning, and she found she was able to be in the present moment when she and Andrew were together (rather than being caught up in her head with mental rituals analyzing their relationship). She found she was able to live her lifewithout a 100% iron-clad guarantee that Andrew was "the one" (and not letting that paralyze her or hold her back). Once Stephanie was better able to tolerate her relationship uncertainty, she found she was in a clearer place to make a values-based decision about the relationship (whereas before her OCD had been obscuring any ability to know her true feelings). Even though ERP had wrapped up by the time Stephanie and Andrew got married, she sent her therapist an email after the ceremony expressing gratitude for ultimately helping them get to the altar.

Case 4: Unacceptable Thoughts About Harm

Greg was a religious 45-year-old elementary school teacher with recurrent unwanted thoughts and images involving being responsible for harming his students (e.g., by stabbing or strangling them). These obsessions were triggered by hearing certain words (e.g., "strangle" or "stab") and by the sight of children – especially the students in his classroom that Greg cared for – which would often trigger horrific images of their dead bodies. In the classroom, Greg tried to keep a distance between himself and any sharp objects (e.g., stapler, scissors, sharp pencils). Greg had even called out sick from work several times recently when he could not bring himself to face these thoughts. He feared that the frequency and intensity of his obsessions indicated that he was truly a danger to his students. When such thoughts came to mind, he tried to analyze their meaning or reassure himself that he would never do such a terrible thing. Greg also prayed ritualistically that he would not harm his students. None of these strategies successfully diminished his obsessions. Greg had no history of engaging in violent behavior and emphatically stated that these thoughts were the exact opposite of how he truly felt towards his students (which was to care for them deeply and want to protect them from harm).

Items on Greg's exposure list included the following (listed here in ascending order of SUDS; Table 11).

Table 11
Greg's Exposure List (With SUDS)

Item	SUDS
Words ("strangle," "stab," and "murderer")	55
Pictures of his classroom of students	65
Movies in which children were harmed	75
News stories in which children were harmed	75
Holding sharp objects and thinking about harming children at home	75
Holding sharp objects and thinking about harming children at school	90
Imaginal exposure to never knowing for sure if he'll one day harm a student	95

Note. SUDS = subjective units of distress.

Greg's response prevention plan was as follows:

- No mental analyzing the meaning of thoughts
- Refrain from any prayers about intrusive thoughts
- No self-reassurance that the thoughts don't mean anything

During the first exposure session, Greg brought a class picture of his students to look at. The therapist asked Greg to allow images of dead bodies to come without trying to fight them. Greg was fearful that he would not be able to keep these images in his mind for very long but was surprised to find that he was able to do so for at least half an hour without praying or ritualizing. Greg was instructed to repeat this exercise each day between sessions, for longer and longer durations, in different places (e.g., home, school classroom, at the playground, etc.).

During the second exposure session, Greg practiced saying the words "strangle," "stab," "murderer," which provoked anxiety for him. He also repeatedly wrote these words on sheets of paper that he kept in his wallet. Homework practice included repeating these exercises daily and discovering that the distress associated with these words was manageable.

At exposure session three, Greg read a news story about a male teacher who was arrested for physically assaulting one of his students. He was instructed to allow himself to acknowledge the similarities between himself and this teacher (e.g., age, gender). He also practiced tolerating uncertainty of not knowing if there might one day be a news article written about him. He repeated this task between sessions, and also found movie clips to watch and book passages to read in which children were harmed. Greg found that the uncertainty evoked by these exercises was more bearable than he had predicted it would be.

At the fourth session, Greg again practiced viewing the class picture of his students, and this time he also wrote a story describing himself suddenly snapping and harming one of them (via strangulation). Greg was instructed to vividly describe the events. He expressed concern that doing so might make him become a murderer; thus, the exposure was engineered to help Greg embrace this uncertainty. Greg's therapist helped him learn that despite the distress he encountered, Greg could remain uncertain, without reassuring himself, analyzing, or praying. Between sessions, Greg wrote similar stories, some of which focused on the worst-case scenario, and some of which focused on never knowing for sure if these feared consequences would one day occur. He practiced thinking about this uncertainty in different contexts as well (e.g., at school) and began listening to them at home while holding sharp objects.

By exposure session five, Greg had made a lot of progress but still reported difficulty refraining from certain mental rituals that were so habitual (e.g., self-reassurance, overanalyzing). Thus, the therapist introduced some mindfulness skills in the session to help Greg get out of his head and into the present moment, to especially be applied in the classroom when he was teaching. Greg practiced these mindfulness exercises daily and found the exercises that involved tolerating unpleasant obsessional thoughts and feelings without needing to fix them were especially helpful. He also benefitted from repeatedly practicing bringing his mind back when it wandered.

Exposure session six was spent planning for a between-session exposure in which Greg would walk around the classroom holding sharp objects that he would typically avoid (e.g., a sharp pencil). Greg planned to allow the harm intrusive thoughts be there without ritualizing. Greg was able to complete this exposure with very few rituals, despite feeling distressed. Although distress level was not used as an indicator of success, Greg found that by the end of the class his fear had substantially reduced. At the following session, the therapist reminded Greg that there was still no guarantee that Greg was not a danger to his students and yet he was able to feel "comfortably uncomfortable." Greg was surprised at this achievement.

The sessions that followed involved repeating the exposure from session six with more challenging objects (e.g., scissors), as well as combining this task with imaginal exposure (i.e., listening to a recording on his lunch break before class and then completing the exercise while purposely conjuring up thoughts of harming his students). By this time, Greg felt comfortable performing exposures on his own and was taking a more active role in designing his own exposures to up the ante.

6

Further Reading

Abramowitz, J. (2006). *Understanding and treating obsessive-compulsive disorder: A cognitive-behavioral approach.* Lawrence Erlbaum. https://doi.org/10.4324/9781410615718
Presents didactic material on the clinical features and psychological theories of OCD. Also contains a manual for cognitive-behavioral assessment and treatment.

Abramowitz, J. S., & Blakey, S. M. (2020). *Clinical handbook of fear and anxiety: Maintenance processes and treatment mechanisms.* American Psychological Association.
Provides an in-depth exploration of the mechanisms that maintain OCD and related anxiety disorders and illustrative descriptions and examples of evidence-based treatment approaches, including exposure, response prevention, cognitive therapy, and ACT.

Abramowitz, J. S., Deacon, B. J., & Whiteside, S. P. (2019). *Exposure therapy for anxiety: Principles and practice* (2nd ed.). Guilford Press.
Offers a detailed guide to the conceptual principles and practical application of exposure therapy for treating anxiety-related disorders, including the various presentations of OCD. The second edition covers various techniques and strategies to help clinicians effectively implement exposure-based treatments from an inhibitory learning perspective.

Arch, J. J., & Abramowitz, J. S. (2015). Exposure therapy for obsessive-compulsive disorder: An optimizing inhibitory learning approach. *Journal of Obsessive-Compulsive and Related Disorders, 6*, 174–182. https://doi.org/10.1016/j.jocrd.2014.12.002
This paper outlines strategies to optimize treatment outcomes by focusing on inhibitory learning mechanisms.

Ferrando, C., & Selai, C. (2021). A systematic review and meta-analysis on the effectiveness of exposure and response prevention therapy in the treatment of obsessive-compulsive disorder. *Journal of Obsessive-Compulsive and Related Disorders, 31*, 1–16. https://doi.org/10.1016/j.jocrd.2021.100684
This systematic review confirms the robust effectiveness of ERP, with significant reductions in symptom severity across studies. ERP consistently outperformed control conditions, including waitlist and placebo, highlighting it as a gold-standard treatment. The authors also noted variability in treatment outcomes and emphasized the need for more research into moderators of ERP effectiveness.

Jacoby, R. J., & Abramowitz, J. S. (2016). Inhibitory learning approaches to exposure therapy: A critical review and translation to obsessive-compulsive disorder. *Clinical Psychology Review, 49*, 28–40. https://doi.org/10.1016/j.cpr.2016.07.001
Examines the application of inhibitory learning principles in ERP for OCD, reviews existing research, and translates these approaches into practical strategies for improving treatment outcomes.

Levy, H. C., O'Bryan, E. M., & Tolin, D. F. (2021). A meta-analysis of relapse rates in cognitive-behavioral therapy for anxiety disorders. *Journal of Anxiety Disorders, 81*, Article 102407. https://doi.org/10.1016/j.janxdis.2021.102407

This study examined relapse rates following CBT for anxiety-related disorders and found that while CBT is highly effective in the short term, relapse is not uncommon over time. The study emphasizes the importance of booster sessions, maintenance strategies, and long-term follow-up to support sustained gains. Relapse rates varied by disorder, with OCD showing relatively lower relapse compared to other anxiety disorders.

Ong, C. W., Clyde, J. W., Bluett, E. J., Levin, M. E., & Twohig, M. P. (2016). Dropout rates in exposure with response prevention for obsessive-compulsive disorder: What do the data really say? *Journal of Anxiety Disorders, 40*, 8–17. https://doi.org/10.1016/j.janxdis.2016.03.006
This paper challenges the assumption that ERP for OCD has unacceptably high dropout rates. By systematically reviewing dropout statistics across studies, the authors found that ERP's dropout rates are around 19% and are comparable to other evidence-based treatments for anxiety-related disorders.

Pinciotti, C. M., Smith, Z., Singh, S., Wetterneck, C. T., & Williams, M. T. (2022). Call to action: Recommendations for justice-based treatment of obsessive-compulsive disorder with sexual orientation and gender themes. *Behavior Therapy, 53*(2), 153–169. https://doi.org/10.1016/j.beth.2021.11.001
This article issues a call to action for justice-based treatment of OCD, particularly for individuals with sexual orientation and gender-related themes in their obsessions. The authors highlight how traditional ERP can inadvertently reinforce stigma or harm if not delivered with cultural humility and affirming practices.

Twohig, M. P., Abramowitz, J. S., Bluett, E. J., Fabricant, L. E., Jacoby, R. J., Morrison, K. L., Reuman, L., & Smith, B. M. (2015). Exposure therapy for OCD from an acceptance and commitment therapy (ACT) framework. *Journal of Obsessive-Compulsive and Related Disorders, 6*, 167–173. https://doi.org/10.1016/j.jocrd.2014.12.007
This paper outlines how combining ACT and ERP can enhance treatment for OCD by fostering psychological flexibility.

Wheaton, M. G., Galfalvy, H., Steinman, S. A., Wall, M. M., Foa, E. B., & Simpson, H. B. (2016). Patient adherence and treatment outcome with exposure and response prevention for OCD: Which components of adherence matter and who becomes well? *Behaviour Research and Therapy, 85*, 6–12. https://doi.org/10.1016/j.brat.2016.07.010
This study explored the role of client adherence in the success of ERP for OCD, finding that higher adherence to both in-session exposures and between-session homework predicted better outcomes. Notably, those who became symptom-free were more likely to have consistently engaged with all components of ERP. The findings underscore the importance of fostering engagement and addressing barriers to adherence to optimize treatment success.

7

References

Abramovitch, A., Abramowitz, J. S., & McKay, D. (2021). The OCI-4: An ultra-brief screening scale for obsessive-compulsive disorder. *Journal of Anxiety Disorders, 78,* Article 102354.

Abramovitch, A., Abramowitz, J. S., & Mittleman, A. (2013). The neuropsychology of adult obsessive-compulsive disorder: A meta-analysis. *Clinical Psychology Review, 33,* 1163–1171. https://doi.org/10.1016/j.cpr.2013.09.004

Abramowitz, J. S. (2025). *Living well with OCD: Practical strategies for improving your daily life*. Guilford Press.

Abramowitz, J. S., Baucom, D. H., Wheaton, M. G., Boeding, S., Fabricant, L. E., Paprocki, C., & Fischer, M. S. (2013). Enhancing exposure and response prevention for OCD: A couple-based approach. *Behavior Modification, 37,* 189–210. https://doi.org/10.1177/0145445512444596

Abramowitz, J. S., Deacon, B., Olatunji, B., Wheaton, M. G., Berman, N., Losardo, D., Timpano, K., McGrath, P., Riemann, B., Adams, T., Bjorgvinsson, T., Storch, E. A., & Hale, L. (2010). Assessment of obsessive-compulsive symptom dimensions: Development and evaluation of the Dimensional Obsessive-Compulsive Scale. *Psychological Assessment, 22,* 180–198. https://doi.org/10.1037/a0018260

Abramowitz, J. S., & Jacoby, R. J. (2014). Scrupulosity: A cognitive–behavioral analysis and implications for treatment. *Journal of Obsessive-Compulsive and Related Disorders, 3*(2), 140–149. https://doi.org/10.1016/j.jocrd.2013.12.007

American Psychiatric Association. (2022). *Diagnostic and statistical manual of mental disorders* (5th ed., text revision).

Brown, T. A., & Barlow, D. H. (2014). *Anxiety and related disorders interview schedule for DSM-5 (ADIS-5)-adult and lifetime version: Clinician manual.* Oxford University Press.

Buchholz, J. L., & Abramowitz, J. S. (2020). The therapeutic alliance in exposure therapy for anxiety-related disorders: A critical review. *Journal of Anxiety Disorders, 70,* 102194. https://doi.org/10.1016/j.janxdis.2020.102194

Buchholz, J. L., Blakey, S. M., Hellberg, S. N., Massing-Schaffer, M., Reuman, L., Ojalehto, H., Friedman, J., & Abramowitz, J. S. (2022). Expectancy violation during exposure therapy: A pilot randomized controlled trial. *Journal of Behavioral and Cognitive Therapy, 32*(1), 13–24. https://doi.org/10.1016/j.jbct.2021.12.004

Clark, D. A., & Radomsky, A. (2014). Introduction: A global perspective on unwanted thoughts. *Journal of Obsessive-Compulsive and Related Disorders, 3*(3), 265–268. https://doi.org/10.1016/j.jocrd.2014.02.001

Craske, M., & Barlow, D. H. (2006). *Mastery of your anxiety and panic (Therapist guide).* Oxford University Press. https://doi.org/10.1093/med:psych/9780195311402.001.0001

Craske, M., Treanor, M., Conway, C., Zbozinek, T., & Vervliet, B. (2014). Maximizing exposure therapy: An inhibitory learning approach. *Behaviour Research and Therapy, 58,* 10–23. https://doi.org/10.1016/j.brat.2014.04.006

Deacon, B. J., & Farrell, N. R. (2013). Therapist barriers in the dissemination of exposure therapy. In E. Storch & D. McKay. (Eds.), *Treating variants and complications in anxiety disorders* (pp. 363–373). Springer Press.

Eisen, J. L., Phillips, K. A., Baer, L., Beer, D. A., Atala, K. D., & Rasmussen, S. A. (1998). The Brown Assessment of Beliefs Scale: Reliability and validity. *American Journal of Psychiatry, 155*(1), 102–108. https://doi.org/10.1176/ajp.155.1.102

Ferrando, C., & Selai, C. (2021). A systematic review and meta-analysis on the effectiveness of exposure and response prevention therapy in the treatment of obsessive-compulsive disorder. *Journal of Obsessive-Compulsive and Related Disorders, 31*, 100684. https://doi.org/10.1016/j.jocrd.2021.100684

First, M. B., Williams, J. B. W., Karg, R. S., & Spitzer, R. L. (2015). Structured Clinical Interview for DSM-5 – Research Version (SCID-5 for DSM-5, Research Version; SCID-5-RV). American Psychiatric Association.

Foa, E. B., Huppert, J. D., & Cahill, S. P. (2006). Emotional processing theory: An update. In B. O. Rothbaum (Ed.), *Pathological anxiety: Emotional processing in etiology and treatment* (pp. 3–24). Guilford Press.

Foa, E., & Kozak, M. (1986). Emotional processing of fear: Exposure to corrective information. *Psychological Bulletin, 99*, 20–35. https://doi.org/10.1037/0033-2909.99.1.20

Foa, E., Liebowitz, M. R., Kozak, M. J., Davies, S., Campeas, R., Franklin, M. E., Huppert, J. D., Kjernisted, K., Rowan, V., Schmidt, A. B., Simpson, H. B., & Tu, X. (2005). Randomized, placebo-controlled trial of exposure and ritual prevention, clomipramine, and their combination in the treatment of obsessive-compulsive disorder. *American Journal of Psychiatry, 162*, 151–161. https://doi.org/10.1176/appi.ajp.162.1.151

Franklin, M. E., Abramowitz, J. S., Foa, E. B., Kozak, M. J., & Levitt, J. T. (2000). Effectiveness of exposure and ritual prevention for obsessive-compulsive disorder: Randomized compared with nonrandomized samples. *Journal of Consulting and Clinical Psychology, 68*(4), 594–602. https://doi.org/10.1037/0022-006X.68.4.594

Frost, R. O., & Steketee, S. (2002). *Cognitive approaches to obsessions and compulsions: Theory, assessment, and treatment.* Elsevier.

Goodman, W. K., Price, L. H., Rasmussen, S. A., Mazure, C., Delgado, P., Heninger, G. R., & Charney, D. S. (1989). The Yale-Brown Obsessive Compulsive Scale: Validity. *Archives of General Psychiatry, 46*, 1012–1016. https://doi.org/10.1001/archpsyc.1989.01810110048007

Goodman, W. K., Price, L. H., Rasmussen, S. A., Mazure, C., Fleischmann, R. L., Hill, C. L., Heninger, G. R., & Charney, D. S. (1989). The Yale-Brown Obsessive Compulsive Scale: Development, use, and reliability. *Archives of General Psychiatry, 46*, 1006–1011. https://doi.org/10.1001/archpsyc.1989.01810110048007

Hassan, W., El Hayek, S., de Filippis, R., Eid, M., Hassan, S., & Shalbafan, M. (2024). Variations in obsessive compulsive disorder symptomatology across cultural dimensions. *Frontiers in Psychiatry, 15*, Article 1329748. https://doi.org/10.3389/fpsyt.2024.1329748

Hayes, S. C., Strosahl, K. D., & Wilson, K. G. (2011). *Acceptance and commitment therapy: The process and practice of mindful change* (2nd ed.). Guilford Press.

Hirschtritt, M. E., Bloch, M. H., Mathews, C. A., & Obsessive-Compulsive Disorder Genetics Collaborative. (2017). Obsessive-compulsive disorder: Advances in diagnosis and treatment. *JAMA, 317*(13), 1358–1367. https://doi.org/10.1001/jama.2017.2200

Hunt, C. (2020). Differences in OCD symptom presentations across age, culture, and gender: A quantitative review of studies using the Y-BOCS symptom checklist. *Journal of Obsessive-Compulsive and Related Disorders, 26*, Article 100533. https://doi.org/10.1016/j.jocrd.2020.100533

Inozu, M., Eremsoy, E., Cicek, N. M., & Ozcanli, F. (2017). The association of scrupulosity with disgust propensity and contamination based obsessive compulsive symptoms: An experimental investigation using highly scrupulous Muslims. *Journal of Obsessive-Compulsive and Related Disorders, 15*, 43-51. https://doi.org/10.1016/j.jocrd.2017.08.004

Jacoby, R. J., & Abramowitz, J. S. (2016). Inhibitory learning approaches to exposure therapy: A critical review and translation to obsessive-compulsive disorder. *Clinical Psychology Review, 49*, 28–40. https://doi.org/10.1016/j.cpr.2016.07.001

Jacoby, R. J., Abramowitz, J. A., Buchholz, J. L., Reuman, L., & Blakey S. M. (2018). Experiential avoidance in the context of obsessions: Development and validation of the Acceptance and Action Questionnaire for Obsessions and Compulsions. *Journal of Obsessive Compulsive and Related Disorders, 19,* 34–43. https://doi.org/10.1016/j.jocrd.2018.07.003

Jacoby, R. J., Smilansky, H., Shin, J., Wu, M. S., Small, B. J., Wilhelm, S., Storch, E. A., & Geller, D. A. (2021). Longitudinal trajectory and predictors of change in family accommodation during exposure therapy for pediatric OCD. *Journal of Anxiety Disorders, 83,* 102463. https://doi.org/10.1016/j.janxdis.2021.102463

Jondani, J. A., Yazdkhasti, F., & Abedi, A. (2023). Memory confidence and memory accuracy deterioration following repeated checking: A systematic review and meta-analysis. *Journal of Behavior Therapy and Experimental Psychiatry, 81,* Article 101855.

Juel, E. K., Rogers, K., Hadlock, S., Myers, N. S., Friedman, J. B., Tadross, M., & Abramowitz, J. S. (2025). An effectiveness study of intensive outpatient treatment for obsessive-compulsive disorder. *Journal of Obsessive-Compulsive and Related Disorders, 44*, 100931.

Kozak, M. J., & Coles, M. E. (2005). Treatment of obsessive-compulsive disorder: Unleashing the power of exposure. In J. S. Abramowitz & A. C. Houts (Eds.), *Concepts and controversies in obsessive-compulsive disorder* (pp. 283–304). Springer.

Lisi, D. M., Hawley, L. L., McCabe, R. E., Rowa, K., Cameron, D. H., Richter, M. A., & Rector, N. A. (2024). Online versus in-person delivery of cognitive behaviour therapy for obsessive compulsive disorder: An examination of effectiveness. *Clinical Psychology & Psychotherapy, 31*(1), e2908. https://doi.org/10.1002/cpp.2908

McKay, D., Abramowitz, J. S., Calamari, J. E., Kyrios, M., Radomsky, A. S., Sookman, D., Taylor, S., & Wilhelm, S. (2004). A critical evaluation of obsessive-compulsive disorder subtypes: Symptoms versus mechanisms. *Clinical Psychology Review, 24*, 283–313. https://doi.org/10.1016/j.cpr.2004.04.003

Mowrer, O. (1960). *Learning theory and behavior.* Wiley. https://doi.org/10.1037/10802-000

Mundt, J. C., Marks, I. M., Shear, M. K., & Greist, J. M. (2002). The Work and Social Adjustment Scale: A simple measure of impairment in functioning. *British Journal of Psychiatry, 180*(5), 461-464. https://doi.org/10.1192/bjp.180.5.461

Obsessive Compulsive Cognitions Working Group. (2005). Psychometric validation of the Obsessive Belief Questionnaire and Interpretation of Intrusions Inventory: Part 2: Factor analyses and testing of a brief version. *Behaviour Research and Therapy, 43*(11), 1527–1542. https://doi.org/10.1016/j.brat.2004.07.010

Olatunji, B., Davis, M., Powers, M., & Smits, J. (2013). Cognitive-behavioral therapy for obsessive-compulsive disorder: A meta-analysis of treatment outcome and moderators. *Journal of Psychiatric Research, 47,* 33–41. https://doi.org/10.1016/j.jpsychires.2012.08.020

Ong, C. W., Clyde, J. W., Bluett, E. J., Levin, M. E., & Twohig, M. P. (2016). Dropout rates in exposure with response prevention for obsessive-compulsive disorder: What do the data really say? *Journal of Anxiety Disorders, 40*, 8–17. https://doi.org/10.1016/j.janxdis.2016.03.006

Pinciotti, C. M., Smith, Z., Singh, S., Wetterneck, C. T., & Williams, M. T. (2022). Call to Action: Recommendations for justice-based treatment of obsessive-compulsive disorder with sexual orientation and gender themes. *Behavior Therapy, 53*(2), 153–169. https://doi.org/10.1016/j.beth.2021.11.001

Rachman, S., & Hodgson, R. (1980). *Obsessions and compulsions*. Prentice Hall.

Radomsky, A. S., Alcolado, G. M., Abramowitz, J. S., Alonso, P., Belloch, A., Bouvard, M., Clark, D. A., Coles, M. E., Doron, G., Fernandez-Alvarez, H., Garcia-Soriano, G., Ghisi, M., Gomez, B., Inozu, M., Moulding, R., Shams, G., Sica, C., & Wong, W.

(2014). Part 1: You can run but you can't hide: Intrusive thoughts on six continents. *Journal of Obsessive-Compulsive and Related Disorders, 3*(3), 269–279. https://doi.org/10.1016/j.jocrd.2013.09.002

Ruscio, A., Stein, D. J., Chiu, D., & Kessler, R. (2010). The epidemiology of obsessive-compulsive disorder in the National Comorbidity Survey Replication. *Molecular Psychiatry, 15*, 53–63. https://doi.org/10.1038/mp.2008.94

Sheehan, D. V., Lecrubier, Y., Harnett-Sheehan, K., Amorim, P., Janavs, J., Weiller, E., Hergueta, T., Baker, R, & Dunbar, G. (1998). The Mini International Neuropsychiatric Interview (M.I.N.I.): The development and validation of a structured diagnostic psychiatric interview. *Journal of Clincial Psychiatry, 59*(Suppl 20), 22–33.

Storch, E. A., De Nadai, A. S., Do Rosário, M. C., Shavitt, R. G., Torres, A. R., Ferrão, Y. A., Miguel, E. C., Lewin, A. B., & Fontenelle, L. F. (2015). Defining clinical severity in adults with obsessive-compulsive disorder. *Comprehensive Psychiatry, 63*, 30–35. https://doi.org/10.1016/j.comppsych.2015.08.007

Swedo, S. E. (2002). Pediatric autoimmune neuropsychiatric disorders associated with streptococcal infections (PANDAS). *Molecular Psychiatry, 7*(2), S24-S25. https://doi.org/10.1038/sj.mp.4001170

Tolin, D. F., Gilliam, C., Wootton, B. M., Bowe, W., Bragdon, L. B., Davis, E., Hannan, S. E., Steinman, S. A., Worden, B., & Hallion, L. S. (2018). Psychometric properties of a structured diagnostic interview for DSM-5 anxiety, mood, and obsessive-compulsive and related disorders. *Assessment, 25*(1), 3–13. https://doi.org/10.1177/1073191116638410

Twohig, M. P., Capel, L. K., & Levin, M. E. (2024). A review of research on acceptance and commitment therapy for anxiety and obsessive-compulsive and related disorders. *Psychiatric Clinics of North America, 47*(4), 711–722. https://doi.org/10.1016/j.psc.2024.04.013

Wheaton, M. G., & Chen, S. R. (2021). Homework completion in treating obsessive-compulsive disorder with exposure and ritual prevention: A review of the empirical literature. *Cognitive Therapy and Research, 45*(2), 236–249. https://doi.org/10.1007/s10608-020-10125-0

Williams, K., Chambless, D. L., & Steketee, G. (1998). Behavioral treatment of obsessive-compulsive disorder in African Americans: Clinical issues. *Journal of Behavior Therapy & Experimental Psychiatry, 29*(2), 163–170. https://doi.org/10.1016/S0005-7916(98)00004-4

Williams, M. T., Rouleau, T. M., La Torre, J. T., & Sharif, N. (2020). Cultural competency in the treatment of obsessive-compulsive disorder: Practitioner guidelines. *The Cognitive Behaviour Therapist, 13*, Article e48. https://doi.org/10.1017/S1754470X20000501

Wilson, A., & Thayer, K. (2020). Cross-cultural differences in the presentation and expression of OCD in Black individuals: A systematic review. *Journal of Obsessive-Compulsive and Related Disorders, 27*, Article 100592. https://doi.org/10.1016/j.jocrd.2020.100592

8

Appendix: Tools and Resources

The following materials for your book can be downloaded free of charge once you register on the Hogrefe website.

Appendix 1: Functional Assessment of OCD Symptoms
Appendix 2: Self-Monitoring of OCD Rituals
Appendix 3: Everyone Has Intrusive Thoughts
Appendix 4: Goal Setting in ERP Worksheet
Appendix 5: Exposure List
Appendix 6: Guidelines for Conducting Exposure
Appendix 7: Exposure Practice Form
Appendix 8: Guidelines for Conducting Imaginal Exposure
Appendix 9: Guidelines for Conducting Response Prevention
Appendix 10: ERP Therapy Summary

How to proceed:

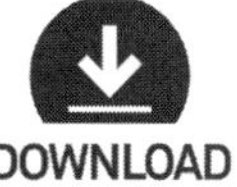

1. Go to www.hgf.io/media and create a user account. If you already have one, please log in.

2. Go to **My supplementary materials** in your account dashboard and enter the code below. You will automatically be redirected to the download area, where you can access and download the supplementary materials.

   Code: B-5RMSIA

To make sure you have permanent direct access to all the materials, we recommend that you download them and save them on your computer.

Appendix 1: Functional Assessment of OCD Symptoms

This is a **preview** of the content that is available in the downloadable material of this book. Please see p. 119 for instructions on how to obtain the full-sized, printable PDF.

Date: ____________________

Client name: ____________________ Present age: ____________________

Date of birth: ____________________ Duration of symptoms: ____________________

Educational level: ____________________

Obsessional Stimuli

- **External triggers of obsessions** (people, places, things, and situations that evoke anxiety; e.g., mold, leaving home, or the number 13)

- **Obsessional thoughts, impulses, images, doubts** (e.g., "God is dead," images of germs, impulse to harm, or doubts about fires)

Cognitive Features

- **Feared consequences of exposure to obsessional triggers** (e.g., "I will get sick if I don't wash my hands")

- **Catastrophic interpretations of intrusive thoughts** (e.g., "Thinking about it is the same as doing it")

- **Fears of long-term anxiety, uncertainty, discomfort, and/or incompleteness** ("I will be anxious forever unless I ritualize" or "I can't tolerate not knowing something for sure")

Responses to Obsessional Distress (Safety-Seeking Behaviors)

- **Passive avoidance** (identify its relationship to obsessional fear; e.g., client avoids old buildings due to fears of asbestos)

- **Overt compulsive rituals** (identify relationships to obsessional fear; e.g., checking the door to prevent burglary; reassurance seeking)

- **Mental rituals, covert neutralizing strategies** (identify relationships to obsessional fear; e.g., suppressing thoughts, mental reviewing, replacing unwanted images with positive images)

Impairment in Quality of Life

- How have you changed your life because of this? How have the obsessions, compulsions, and/or avoidance gotten in the way?

This is a **preview** of the content that is available in the downloadable material of this book. Please see p. 119 for instructions on how to obtain the full-sized, printable PDF.

Appendix 2: Self-Monitoring of OCD Rituals

This is a **preview** of the content that is available in the downloadable material of this book. Please see p. 119 for instructions on how to obtain the full-sized, printable PDF.

Ritual 1: ______________________ Ritual 2: ______________________

Date	Time	What triggered the ritual? (Brief summary of situation or thought)	Distress (SUDS: 0–100)	Minutes spent on ritual		What was the result on your quality of life?
				1	2	

Appendix 3: Everyone Has Intrusive Thoughts

This is a **preview** of the content that is available in the downloadable material of this book. Please see p. 119 for instructions on how to obtain the full-sized, printable PDF.

In obsessive-compulsive disorder (OCD), obsessions are unwanted intrusive thoughts, ideas, or images that cause anxiety, fear, disgust, guilt, "not just right" feelings, uncertainty, and discomfort. These obsessions often seem senseless or bizarre and can involve themes such as harm, violence, aggression, sex, religion, mistakes, physical appearance, germs, diseases, and a need for exactness. Because obsessions cause distress, people try to resist, stop, control, or seek reassurance about these thoughts, but these efforts are often ineffective. As a result, the thoughts return and can seem to take on a "life of their own."

What many people don't realize is that almost everyone experiences unwanted intrusive thoughts, whether or not they have OCD. These thoughts are as normal as fantasies and daydreams about positive events. This handout aims to teach you that the unpleasant, distressing, bizarre, and senseless thoughts you're experiencing are not dangerous or abnormal.

Intrusive Thoughts Are Normal

Everyone experiences senseless intrusive thoughts and doubts. Whether it's a daydream about winning the lottery, a frightening image of harm, a senseless idea that contradicts your usual thinking or values, or existential uncertainty about the meaning of life, all humans have nonsensical and unwanted thoughts and doubts. You might be surprised to learn that nearly everyone has intrusive, upsetting, and inappropriate thoughts similar to those seen in OCD. Here are some examples of unwanted intrusive thoughts reported by people *without* OCD:

- Thought of jumping off a bridge
- Thought of running a car off the road
- Thought of poking something into my eyes
- Impulse to jump onto the tracks as a train comes
- Image of hurting a loved one
- Idea of doing something mean to an elderly person or baby
- Thought of wishing someone would die
- Impulse to slap someone
- Thought of something going wrong due to my mistake
- Thought of accidentally hitting someone with my car
- Image of a loved one being injured or killed
- Thought of receiving news of a relative's death
- Idea that others might think I'm guilty of stealing
- Thought of being trapped in a car underwater
- Thought of catching diseases from a toilet
- Thought of dirt always on my hands
- Urge to yell at or insult a friend for no reason
- Impulse to do something shameful or terrible
- Thought that I left a door unlocked
- Thought of my house being broken into while I'm not at home
- Thought that I left an appliance on and will cause a fire
- Thought of sexually molesting young children
- Thought contrary to my moral and religious beliefs
- Hoping someone doesn't succeed
- Thought that I don't love my partner enough
- Thoughts about the vastness of the universe
- Idea that we can never understand the meaning of life

- Thoughts of smashing a table of glass crafts
- Thoughts of violence in sex
- Thought of "unnatural" sexual acts
- Image of a penis
- Image of grandparents having sex
- Thought about objects not arranged perfectly

Why does everyone have these kinds of intrusive thoughts? Probably because humans have highly developed and creative brains that can imagine all sorts of scenarios. Sometimes, our *thought generator* produces thoughts about danger even when no real threat is present. Humans think constantly while awake and even while asleep, so it's expected that our brains sometimes create bizarre or senseless thoughts, or *mental noise*. These thoughts can be triggered by real situations like driving, seeing a weapon, using the bathroom, hearing words related to sex, or seeing a religious icon. Sometimes, they come from out of the blue.

Studies have shown that people with and without OCD have the same kinds of intrusive thoughts. In one well-known study, researchers asked people with and without OCD to list some of their unwanted thoughts. The lists, which looked like the examples you just read, were given to experienced mental health professionals who tried to determine which thoughts came from people with and without OCD. Most of the time, even the professionals couldn't tell the difference. This study, and others like it, confirm that people with OCD don't have something wrong with their brains that causes obsessive thoughts. Instead, obsessions in OCD develop from normal experiences.

Differences Between "Normal" Intrusive Thoughts and "OCD" Obsessions

Even though the *content* of "normal" intrusive thoughts and OCD obsessions are similar, there are other important differences:

1. OCD obsessions are more distressing than normal intrusive thoughts.
2. OCD obsessions are resisted more strongly than normal intrusive thoughts.
3. OCD obsessions are more repetitive than normal intrusive thoughts.

The rest of this handout will explain these differences so you can understand how distressing, recurring, and intense OCD obsessions develop from normal intrusive thoughts.

Why Are OCD Obsessions Distressing?

Although everyone has unwanted intrusive thoughts, people interpret these thoughts differently. When these thoughts are seen as especially threatening, they cause fear, anxiety, and distress. People without OCD usually regard these thoughts as "mental noise" and recognize them as meaningless. They might say to themselves, "That's a silly thought," or "That doesn't make sense," and the thought might pass or even linger, without causing distress.

People with OCD, however, misinterpret these thoughts as meaningful, significant, threatening, or dangerous, and needing control. For example:

- "It is bad to have this kind of thought."
- "If I am thinking something bad, it must be true."
- "If I think of something awful, it means I am an awful person."
- "If I have bad thoughts, it means I am losing my mind or will do something terrible."
- "I need to get rid of these thoughts."

This type of interpretation makes the thought seem threatening, and makes the person feel distressed and anxious. But the real problem is the interpretation of the intrusive thought, not the thought itself. Misinterpreting normal intrusive thoughts as significant or dangerous turns them into distressing preoccupations.

This is a **preview** of the content that is available in the downloadable material of this book. Please see p. 119 for instructions on how to obtain the full-sized, printable PDF.

Why Are OCD Obsessions Resisted?

Misinterpreting certain unwanted thoughts as dangerous leads to distress and a desire to resist or push the thought out of your mind. If someone believes an intrusive thought is threatening, significant, important, or dangerous, they will naturally try to push it away.

Why Are OCD Obsessions Repetitive?

The repetitiveness of obsessions is also related to how a person interprets their unwanted thoughts. Once an intrusive thought is seen as threatening, it activates the body's fight-or-flight response, which is the automatic danger detection system, causing hyperalertness and preoccupation with the thought, causing it to become repetitive.

Other responses to intrusive thoughts, such as thought suppression, can increase the repetitiveness of obsessions. Trying to push unwanted thoughts out of your mind often leads to an increase in those thoughts. This is a normal phenomenon – just try not to think of a pink elephant (before you know it, thoughts of pink elephants will be there that weren't before!). Misinterpreted intrusive thoughts, seen as dangerous, lead to futile attempts to suppress them, creating a vicious cycle of anxiety and more unwanted thoughts.

A useful phrase that illustrates this is "If you don't want it, you'll have it." This means that trying to control, resist, or dismiss obsessional thoughts only makes you more preoccupied with them.

Conclusions

Everyone has intrusive, unwanted, upsetting thoughts from time to time. These thoughts, and the anxiety, disgust, and doubt they cause, are normal. They do not indicate danger, evil, ungodliness, perversion, or immorality. They are simply senseless thoughts. The major difference between people with and without OCD is how they relate to and interpret these thoughts. People with OCD see their thoughts as significant, meaningful, and dangerous, leading to anxiety and distress. Treatment for OCD aims to help you see these thoughts as "mental noise" so that when they appear, they don't drive you to engage in compulsive rituals.

This is a **preview** of the content that is available in the downloadable material of this book. Please see p. 119 for instructions on how to obtain the full-sized, printable PDF.

Appendix 4: Goal Setting in ERP Worksheet

This is a **preview** of the content that is available in the downloadable material of this book. Please see p. 119 for instructions on how to obtain the full-sized, printable PDF.

Everyone has their own goals for treatment. Here, write down your goals. Be specific and concrete so you know just what they are. What would that look like? How would you know when you've gotten there? This way, you will be able to keep your eye on the prize and know how well you are progressing toward your goals throughout treatment.

#1: How do you want your obsessional thoughts to be different or improve? (e.g., these could be about wanting to be more in the present moment or to be better at managing anxiety, uncertainty, and doubt)

1. ______
2. ______
3. ______
4. ______

#2: How do you want your compulsive behaviors to be different or improve? (e.g., to reduce time spent on compulsions)

1. ______
2. ______
3. ______
4. ______

#3: How do you want your quality of life to be different or improve? (for this section, consider how you might reduce avoidance, re-engage with social and recreational activities, and/or improve your relationships)

1. ______
2. ______
3. ______
4. ______

Appendix 5: Exposure List

This is a **preview** of the content that is available in the downloadable material of this book. Please see p. 119 for instructions on how to obtain the full-sized, printable PDF.

Items	SUDS
1.	
2.	
3.	
4.	
5.	
6.	
7.	
8.	
9.	
10.	
11.	
12.	
13.	
14.	
15.	
16.	
17.	
18.	
19.	
20.	

Appendix 6: Guidelines for Conducting Exposure

This is a **preview** of the content that is available in the downloadable material of this book. Please see p. 119 for instructions on how to obtain the full-sized, printable PDF.

1. **Exposure practices should be structured.** Prepare for the exercise in advance (as needed) to make sure that it is conducted properly and that you have any materials you might need. Decide what you will do in the situation and how long you will stay. Plan when you will complete your practice and put it in your schedule. Have a back-up plan in case the original does not work out.
2. **Exposure practices should be repeated frequently and in different contexts.** Practice the same exposure tasks multiple times and under different conditions to maximize learning.
3. **Vary up your exposure practices.** Push yourself to practice exposures in a random order – not simply starting with the easiest situations and going gradually. Decide on exposure tasks based on your life values or pick them at random. Challenge yourself!
4. **Expect to feel uncomfortable.** Exposure tasks typically evoke discomfort. This discomfort, however, is necessary for you to learn how to handle obsessions in a healthier way. And whether or not it subsides as you remain in the exposure, you will learn something important. Success should not be judged by how you felt in the situation. Rather, success should be judged by whether you were able to stay in the situation *despite* feeling anxious.
5. **Try not to fight your fear.** Anxiety and fear are the raw materials of change. You will not benefit from exposure if you fight them. Instead of trying to make anxiety, uncertainty, disgust, and distress *go away*, you are learning to be *better* at having these feelings.
6. **Don't use subtle avoidance strategies.** Complete exposure practices without using distraction, thought suppression, antianxiety medication, alcohol, and other such anxiety-reduction strategies.
7. **Use exposure practices to test negative predictions about the consequences of facing your fear.** Before starting the exposure, think about what you are afraid might happen during the task and how long you can stick with it. Then conduct the exposure practice to test the accuracy of your fearful prediction. Afterwards, review what you learned from the exposure and how it compares with what you expected. Did the worst possible thing happen? How did you manage?
8. **Keep track of your fear level.** Pay attention to how you are feeling during the exposure task. Take note of your anxiety level at regular intervals and rate your fear level from 0–100. This will teach you that you can manage different levels of anxiety.
9. **Exposure should last until you have tested a prediction.** Continue the exposure until you have demonstrated that what you feared is unlikely to happen, or that you can handle feelings of anxiety and uncertainty about your obsessions. Try to surprise yourself with what you learn from exposures.
10. **Practice exercises by yourself.** It is helpful to conduct some exposures by yourself because the presence of other people can sometimes make us feel artificially safe. You can do this!

Appendix 7: Exposure Practice Form

This is a **preview** of the content that is available in the downloadable material of this book. Please see p. 119 for instructions on how to obtain the full-sized, printable PDF.

Date: ____________________ Time: ____________________

Check one: ______ Alone ______ Accompanied

Before you start

1. Describe the exposure (What fears will you approach and what distress-reduction strategies will you give up?)

   ____

   ____

   ____

   ____

2. What do you most fear will happen when you try this exposure (be specific)?

   ____

   ____

   ____

   ____

3. What are your goals? How long do you think you can stick with this task?

   ____

   ____

During the exposure

1. Every ______ minutes during the exposure note (a) your distress level and (b) the strength of your urge to do distress-reducing behaviors on a 0–100 scale.

Distress	Urge	Distress	Urge	Distress	Urge	Distress	Urge
1. ___		6. ______	________	11 ______	________	16. ______	________
2. ______	________	7. ______	________	12. ______	________	17. ______	________
3. ______	________	8. ______	________	13. ______	________	18. ______	________
4. ______	________	9. ______	________	14. ______	________	19. ______	________
5. ______	________	10. ______	________	15. ______	________	20. ______	________

2. Describe your feelings during the exposure (use phrases like "I'm feeling very scared about...")

____

____

____

____

After the exposure

1. Describe the outcome of the exposure in relation to your answers to questions #2 and #3 in the "Before" exposure section (What happened? Did you reach your goals? Did your fears come true? How did your feelings of fear and anxiety respond? How did you get through the experience? What would happen if you tried it again?):

____

____

____

____

____

____

2. What did you learn from this experience? In what ways were you surprised by what happened?

____

____

____

____

____

____

3. What could you do to change or vary up this exposure (e.g., different stimuli, up the ante)?

____

____

____

____

____

____

This is a **preview** of the content that is available in the downloadable material of this book. Please see p. 119 for instructions on how to obtain the full-sized, printable PDF.

Appendix 8: Guidelines for Conducting Imaginal Exposure

This is a **preview** of the content that is available in the downloadable material of this book. Please see p. 119 for instructions on how to obtain the full-sized, printable PDF.

1. **Write in the first person:** For example, write, "I accidentally leave the stove on when I go to work" rather than "She left the stove on." These scripts are intended to be personalized about *you*.
2. **Write in the present tense:** Write the scenario like it is unfolding now (e.g., "As I leave my apartment" vs. "When I left my apartment").
3. **Keep it realistic:** Try and make the scenario as lifelike as possible. It must be believable to be effective. If the script becomes too fantastical it will be less useful. Use specifics like people's names (e.g., "Christina" rather than "my girlfriend" or "someone") to make the script feel even more real.
4. **Keep it succinct:** Imaginal exposures scripts should be relatively short and to the point – typically no more than one half to three quarters of a page. No need for extra setup or background; just stick to the content of what upsets you the most. Also, refrain from incorporating your compulsions into your script (e.g., "I reassure myself that I would never really do this") as this can serve to artificially lower your anxiety just like real compulsions.
5. **Take it to the max:** Include all the parts that are the most difficult for you to think about (i.e., your worst fears happening or never knowing for sure if they one day will). For example, perhaps the scenario ends with you spending the rest of your life in prison for murder or having to be uncertain about a feared outcome forever (e.g., "I'll never know for sure if I will one day snap and stab someone"). Focus on the parts that you feel responsible for (e.g., you were the last one to leave the house and are responsible for the apartment complex burning down). By facing your fears directly, you're taking some of the power back that these thoughts currently have over you.
6. **Include all the details:**
   - What are your surroundings? What do you see? Who are you with? (e.g., "I see the flames and smoke billowing from the burning building")
   - What do you hear? Smell? Touch? (e.g., "I hear the screams of the bystanders")
   - What thoughts are going through your mind? (e.g., "I can't believe what I have done")
   - How do you feel emotionally? (e.g., "I'm frozen with fear")
   - What bodily sensations or physical reactions do you experience? (e.g., "I feel sick to my stomach")
   - What behavioral urges do you have? How do you react behaviorally? (e.g., "I feel a strong urge to ask for reassurance, but I know I'll never know the answer for sure")
7. **Read the script repeatedly:** Read the script out loud repeatedly and/or audio record it and listen over and over. Just as you need to repeat situational exposures to learn from them, you will need to repeat imaginal exposures many times to see the most benefit. While of course you will never be comfortable with the feared consequences in the script *actually* occurring, the goal is to read the imaginal exposure until the thoughts alone do not "boss you around" the way they do now, and you learn that you are able to tolerate these thoughts and they don't deserve as much attention and distress.
8. **No skimming:** The goal is to feel the impact of the story and allow your fears to fully sink in, not to get through it as quickly as possible.
9. **Watch out for subtle mental rituals:** For instance, you might find yourself engaging in self-reassurance that this scenario will never happen. When you notice these behaviors, guide yourself back to sticking with the script and focusing on the uncertainty.
10. **Combine with situational exposure:** For example, you can combine reading your imaginal exposure script with looking at a photo of the person you are afraid you will harm or listening to the recording in a real-world situation (e.g., with the person you are worried about harming nearby).
11. **Use this skill in the future:** If a new obsession appears in the future, write a new script. The sooner you tackle the new obsession head on, the less likely it is to get stuck in your mind.

Appendix 9: Guidelines for Response Prevention

This is a **preview** of the content that is available in the downloadable material of this book. Please see p. 119 for instructions on how to obtain the full-sized, printable PDF.

The fastest way to see a reduction in your OCD symptoms is to eliminate rituals completely once you've done an exposure exercise (e.g., once you've done an exposure to leaving the house without checking the stove, refraining from all stove checking). However, for some clients with OCD this may not be possible right away for everyone. Here are some additional strategies you can use to reduce OCD rituals over time:

1. **Stimulus Control:** Manipulate your environment to make it more difficult for the ritual to occur. Deliberately (but temporarily!) avoid certain situations, activities, or objects that trigger or increase rituals. Just be sure to approach these triggers again as you progress through treatment. For example temporarily:
   - Stop carrying hand sanitizer with you.
   - Keep your bathroom door closed (or locked) so you are less tempted to wash your hands.
   - Put your cell phone across the room so you are less likely to send a text message asking for reassurance.
2. **Selective Response Prevention:** Initially allow yourself to engage in rituals only in certain situations, but not in others. Pick your battles! You might decide to decrease rituals first that are interfering the most in your life. For example:
   - Allow yourself to check if the door is locked before bed but not before leaving for the day (if you are having trouble getting out of the house in the morning).
   - Start by limiting handwashing at work (but not at home).
3. **Decrease the Time Spent Ritualizing:** Gradually reduce the amount of time spent on rituals. You can also reduce number of repetitions of a given ritual.
   - Decrease shower length by 10 minutes each day.
   - Take one shower per day instead of two.
   - Set a 5-minute timer for checking the stove; leave the kitchen as soon as the timer goes off, whether you are ready to stop checking or not.
   - Limit asking your partner if they saw you hit something while driving to two questions per day.
   - Decrease rituals from 2 hours, to 60 min, to 30 min, 15 min, to 5 min, etc.
4. **Postpone Rituals:** Delay rituals for as long as possible. This is a time when procrastination is a good thing!
   - Postpone checking to see if you uploaded your assignment correctly for 30 minutes (then see if you can go another 30 minutes – you might find the urge to ritualize has decreased!)
5. **Competing Actions:** These are healthy behaviors or activities done to replace rituals that are physically incompatible with the rituals themselves. In social situations they should also be discreet. Competing responses should focus on the same muscle groups used in the compulsions.
   - If you have the urge to tap or touch certain objects to prevent bad things from happening, make a fist or put your hands in your pocket when you have the urge.
6. **Re-approach:** Deliberately re-approach the situation that evoked the ritual.
   - If you washed your hands because you felt dirty after touching your cell phone; touch your cell phone again without washing your hands.
   - After washing your hands after using the bathroom, touch something you feel is contaminated (e.g., your backpack).
   - If you automatically engaged in a mental ritual (like reassuring yourself or replacing a "bad thought" with a "good thought") remind yourself of the uncertainty (i.e., "I can never know for sure") or think the unwanted thought again.

Appendix 10: ERP Therapy Summary

This is a **preview** of the content that is available in the downloadable material of this book. Please see p. 119 for instructions on how to obtain the full-sized, printable PDF.

Lessons learned in treatment to remember (main take-home points)

1. __________

2. __________

3. __________

Long-term goals and steps to achieve them

1. __________

2. __________

3. __________

Potential triggers for symptoms worsening to watch out for

1. __________

2. __________

3. __________

Warning signs that more formal skills may be needed (how would you know things weren't going as well?)

1. __________

2. __________

3. __________

Skills to reimplement as needed in the future (if you were having a more difficult time, what would you do?)

1. __________

2. __________

3. __________

Peer Commentaries

This thoroughly updated second edition offers mental health professionals a clear, concise, evidence-based roadmap for treating OCD in adults. By blending exposure and response prevention with fresh insights from cognitive therapy, ACT, couples therapy, and inhibitory learning, it empowers clinicians to deliver care that is both compassionate and uniquely suited to each client. Rich with expanded clinical guidance, practical tools, and new illustrative case examples, this book stands out as a practical companion for any therapist or trainee seeking confidence and expertise in managing OCD using the latest advances in cognitive behavioral approaches.

Reid Wilson, PhD, Founder and Director, anxieties.com; Author, *Stopping the Noise in Your Head*

Drs. Abramowitz and Jacoby, leaders in the field of OCD, have successfully crafted a user-friendly text for mental health professionals that discusses the nature of OCD, and its evidence-based assessment and treatment. Best practice approaches for assessment and treatment are thoughtfully conveyed with case examples that bring the material to life. This book will be a game changer for those who want to develop their expertise in working with individuals with OCD.

Eric Storch, PhD, Vice Chair & Head of Psychology, Baylor College of Medicine, Houston, TX

In the OCD specialty world, we are often reminded of how lucky we are as clinicians to work with this population and do so using an approach to treatment that really works. Not only does the research repeatedly confirm the efficacy of cognitive behavioral therapy, but if one understands the mechanisms that allow OCD to cause suffering, then CBT with exposure and response prevention simply makes sense to reduce that suffering. In this second edition of Abramowitz and Jacoby's Obsessive-Compulsive Disorder in Adults, *the authors give a thorough and methodical, yet thankfully easy-to-digest presentation of how CBT with ERP can work in practice. The clinical vignettes and clinical "pearls" scattered throughout the book are especially helpful for understanding the* how, *and not just the what and why of OCD treatment. I found myself not only validated for the way I treat OCD and train others to do so, but motivated to try harder to help patients see how capable they really are of mastering this condition.*

Jon Hershfield, MFT, Director, The Center for OCD and Anxiety at Sheppard Pratt; Author, *When a Family Member Has OCD;* Coauthor, *The Mindfulness Workbook for OCD*